The Joy of Being

The Joy of Being

Advanced Kum Nye Practices for Relaxation, Integration & Concentration

Tarthang Tulku

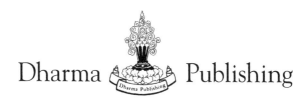

Dharma Publishing

Printed in the U.S.A. at Dharma Mangalam Press
Ratna Ling, California.

Cover and layout design by Ana Paula Wrobel

ISBN: 9780898000849
Library of Congress Control Number: 2016934547

10 9 8 7 6 5 4 3

*Dedicated to experienced Kum Nye
practitioners and teachers around the world.*

*May they achieve special success with the advanced
practices presented in this book.
May they find inner joy, peace, and meaning
as they become masters of Kum Nye.*

Contents

Contents

Contents

PART FIVE: ADVANCED KUM NYE EXERCISES

Contents

Contents

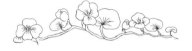

Introduction

Kum (sKu) refers to the body, in the sense of embodied being. Its significance goes beyond our physical form to encompass all aspects of our being and ways we can develop and nurture ourselves as embodiments of authentic existence. Nye (mNye) means massage, or exercise that heals, integrates, and invigorates. Together, the words Kum Nye refer to massage, postures, and exercises that enable us to be comfortable in our embodiment and inspired to awaken the full capacities of body and mind, senses and heart.

The physical exercises of Kum Nye are only the outward forms of a holistic vision of human being. Their true value lies in their ability to stimulate energy that joins body and mind in a continuum of joy and appreciation. In mastering Kum Nye, we learn how to benefit from all manner of experience; we gain confidence that is grounded in self-knowledge and establish a foundation of joy that can sustain us throughout our lives. We learn what it means to be complete in ourselves: We discover what it means to BE.

Kum Nye was known in the time of the early disciples of the Buddha and was continued by later yogic practitioners. In Tibet, it was not always common. In the West, it is best known as a way of massage, but it also includes simple postures and stretches that are yogic in nature, with the main tuning taking place internally.

Exercises presented in the earlier Kum Nye book, *Kum Nye - A Tibetan Yoga, Parts I and II* (Berkeley: Dharma Publishing, 1978, revised 2007), focused on the physical aspects of our being, using massage, breathing exercises, postures, and movement to relax and energize our bodies. *The Joy of Being* goes more deeply into the inner aspects of our embodiment. It emphasizes the inner massage of feeling, using the senses to revitalize our capacities for seeing, hearing, sensing, touching, relishing, and cognizing and creates the basis for a satisfying and meaningful life. It is intended to help you feel at home in your embodiment, so you will appreciate your inner treasures and be inspired to cultivate them further.

Since anyone can begin to develop these treasures without much philosophy or theory, Kum Nye is an effective way to engage meditation. Relaxation that allows the heart to open and meditation to manifest naturally is especially helpful for Western practitioners. As you practice these exercises, senses, mind, and consciousness become more familiar with bliss—the rich nectar of energy flowing unobstructed through a completely relaxed and balanced body. Bliss heals the heart beset by anxiety and pain and restores calm to the pressured and conflicted mind. When bliss becomes part of your being, mind and body will cooperate when you wish to meditate, and you will no longer have to struggle so much with physical and mental distractions. So before you meditate, relax deeply and use Kum Nye to touch blissful states. Once bliss has served its purpose, you can let it go and rest in the relaxed calmness of meditation. If you become attached to bliss and become reluctant to let it go, you will need to find a qualified teacher to help you move beyond it into the deeper current of samadhi.

Kum Nye's way of relaxing body, senses, and mind can introduce us to the power and beauty of the spiritual path. Abundance of joy inspires generosity of heart and the wish to bring joy to others. Joy builds on joy: Joyful in our own being, we take delight in the positive accomplishments of others and spontaneously feel their joy as our own. The suffering of others hits the heart more directly, inspiring compassion and the wish for knowledge that heals and inspires. Love moves beyond self and obligation to manifest more broadly in our actions, and joy stabilizes into equanimity that removes fear and empowers commitment. In this way, the benefits of practicing Kum Nye can transcend the limits of our specific embodiment and generate merit that uplifts all beings.

The Need to BE

Generally, our inability to feel complete in ourselves, to simply BE, compels us to spend much of our time looking for something in a restless, hungry way—friends, distractions, comfort, entertainment—even knowledge. However we might rationalize our motivations, the cause of this restlessness can often be traced to a lack of satisfaction. Most of us eventually reach the point where we realize that something is missing in our lives.

Kum Nye can balance, integrate, and energize the whole of our being, opening clearer channels of communication between senses, body, and mind and inviting a sense of wholeness and calm that is deeply refreshing. When all aspects of our being coexist harmoniously, each supporting and complementing the other, our inner environment becomes happier; our feeling-tones are more generally light and joyful, and our interactions with others are more consistently pleasant. When body and mind are in perfect balance, we are whole and complete: nothing is missing. It is here we may respond to a new vision of human destiny and take the next steps on our spiritual path.

The body, the vehicle that supports and sustains our life, is our most intimate friend, and we need to do all we can to make it more healthy and happy. The mind is also our constant companion; whatever it feels, we feel also, so it is a special pleasure to nourish it with bliss. If you ask, "How is it possible for us to give bliss to our minds at will?" The answer is as close to us as our own bodies, breath, and senses. We can act now to attune the eyes to beauty, the ears to the quality of sound, the nose and tongue to the subtleties of fragrance and taste, and the body to its own vital energy. Then the senses can bring light and joy to the mind dulled with boredom or bound up with negative thoughts and emotions. The mind becomes joyful, awareness expands, and negativity loses its hold. When the mind is content, even the ego becomes mellow; free of the need to protect, assert itself, and defend, it develops the beauty of humility.

Kum Nye can be your gift to yourself, your gesture of gratitude for your embodiment and all the cells and systems that enable you to experience the joy of being alive. Since everyone needs happiness and relief from the frustrations of a busy and often meaningless life, I hope you will make efforts on the behalf of others and dedicate joy to them also. Doing this will greatly magnify the benefits of your efforts.

If you integrate Kum Nye into your daily routine, you can do many of its postures and exercises as you go about your daily activities, during short breaks from work, and in morning and evening. Then, when you meet with difficult times, you will have knowledge and techniques that will help you cope more effectively.

Whatever your activities, you may someday learn that it is possible to have a more flexible way of being. If you develop your sensory capacities, you may come to view your daily activities in a more aesthetic light. If you give joy to your mind, you may find ways to transform your attitudes and apply new knowledge and techniques that bring ease to daily life and work. Whatever you do can become an exercise in Kum Nye, stimulating imagination and creativity.

This book is my way of sharing my thoughts with you. For a long time, I have been considering how to present the more advanced aspects of Kum Nye in a practical way that can benefit individuals in their daily lives and also support those who wish to engage more profound meditative states. Recently, I worked with Elizabeth Cook to compile my ideas into this book, and added exercises designed to convey a sense of the physical, sensory, and mental experiences possible through Kum Nye.

While some orientation is helpful, words alone cannot connect you with Kum Nye: it is the practice that gives you the direct experience, and it is the experience that enables you to transform the quality of your life. Since the benefits of Kum Nye accumulate with regular practice, it is important that you select four to five exercises from this volume about every three months and remind yourself to practice one or two of them at least twice daily. In all you do, remember that Kum Nye is your armament against negativity that scratches from within or affects you through others. It is knowledge that you can master and sustain through mindfulness.

Eventually, when you are familiar with the Kum Nye way of intensifying feelings and sensations, you will not need any reminder—relaxation will come naturally, because you embody the knowledge and attitudes cultivated through Kum Nye. Whatever you are looking for—power, positive feelings, a companion, or love—these are nothing in comparison to the richness of spirit Kum Nye can provide. There is no need to renounce or to give up what you cherish. You can accommodate all manifestations of mind and make joy out of whatever you do.

Your body/mind embodiment is your personal treasure house, a source of beautiful feelings and profound satisfaction. If you appreciate its value and learn how to nurture it well, Kum Nye will show you how to enter the heart of your being and cultivate your inner riches more fully. Kum Nye will awaken the joy of being; Kum Nye will bring you home.

Introduction

Kum Nye - A Tibetan Yoga has been published around the world in fifteen languages and a photobook edition entitled *Tibetan Relaxation* has been issued in English, Dutch, French, German, and Portuguese. I hope *The Joy of Being* inspires new practitioners and encourages experienced ones to allow Kum Nye to touch their hearts more directly. May these essays inspire your practice and ease your journey through life.

Tarthang Tulku
Odiyan, August 1, 2005

Preface to the 3rd Edition

I am very pleased to write this preface for the third edition of The Joy of Being. I took quite a different approach in this book than I did in my earlier books on Kum Nye. In The Joy of Being, instead of focusing on a more traditional graduated set of exercises, I first emphasize how to embody Kum Nye—how to be present within the present.

In particular, Part Three, which introduces the sense faculties, gives readers ways to explore what is taking place when we see, hear, smell, taste, feel or think. The layers that open up when we examine our senses more closely can enable us to perceive new and different dimensions of the experience of being.

For our senses are sources of precious treasures. Through them, we can experience states of bliss and wonder so refined that they have no names. Our embodiment as human beings is an incredible opportunity to discover a subtle, transformative knowledge, a joy far beyond conditions and boundaries.

This joy is our birthright. If we can understand how it arises, we have a resource we can rely upon no matter what comes; this treasure cannot be taken from us. But since understanding plays a crucial role in whether we have access to this treasure, ultimately the main emphasis of this book is on Kum Nye for the mind.

In *The Joy of Being* you will find several ways that Kum Nye's power of relaxation can help melt the tensions embedded in the words "I," "me" and "mine." Kum Nye relaxes the regime of mind; it has the potential to bring forth a quality of shining openness that gives mind time and space to *BE*. New powers of mind naturally emerge, and we discover that in our nature, we are already complete: there is nothing missing.

The light of this awareness has the potential to illuminate our spiritual path. It can guide us in our attitudes, in how we speak, and how we act. In this way, we can make conscious contact with our innermost selves, and taste true happiness.

It is so important to embody happiness. If we cannot take responsibility for our experience and cultivate our joy, we cannot be our best selves. It is when we are able to make the most of our experiences that we can truly bring joy to others.

Please read this book a few times, slowly and meditatively, giving yourself the chance to digest what it says. Give yourself the gift of time to practice, to absorb and learn, so that your precious inheritance, your human embodiment, does not remain a hidden treasure. Practice regularly; encourage yourself through your experiences.

You, yourself, can discover the meaning of being, the meaning of joy.

Tarthang Tulku
Odiyan, February 23, 2016

How to Use This Book: A Message from the Editor

The essays and exercises in this book are organized under four major headings: The Working Basis, Breath, Senses and Perception, and Massaging Mind. Although the order of topics and exercises is not necessarily progressive, you are advised to read the book through from cover to cover before selecting an area of focus. It is helpful to view this entire book as exercises for the mind.

Sensory perception is an important and complex study that is explored in great detail in Buddhist treatises on Abhidharma. Also, where Western systems make distinctions between the physical senses and mind, Buddhist traditions generally group together the physical senses and the sensing aspect of mind, forming a total of six senses. Sensing is but one aspect of mind as mind is understood in the West. Buddhist Abhidharma systems go on to name different aspects of mind, define the operation of each one, and distinguish different levels of consciousness.

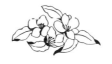

Kum Nye is our greatest treasure, a right to be cultivated and embodied, a heritage to be revitalized and expressed through our attitudes and actions. It is because of the knowledge preserved within Kum Nye that the Buddha is a symbol of universal peace and the Dharma is a symbol of healing and transformation. We cannot let this knowledge die.

—Tarthang Tulku

Part One

The Working Basis

In all this world, there is nothing more important than appreciating the preciousness of our human embodiment and doing all we can to increase health and happiness for ourselves and others.

Those of us caught in the confusing currents of modern life may tend to set aside this priority until we become ill or exhausted. But here is where Kum Nye can be most helpful. Its exercises awaken the knowledge we need to enrich our lives and benefit all of humanity, yet they also fit easily into our daily routines. If you love yourself, if you love others, the rewards of practicing Kum Nye will be greater than you can imagine.

So it is important to make strong efforts to develop this knowledge and apply it. You can do this by reminding yourself daily: There is beauty that you have not yet seen. There is sound that carries consciousness into heavenly spheres. There is fragrance more exquisite than the rarest incense. There is joy that expands beyond ecstasy and dissolves the seeds of suffering. You deserve to experience all these treasures and manifest their significance to all humanity.

1

Kum Nye is Life

Kum Nye is a way to relax body and mind, to awaken the senses, to nurture ourselves with enjoyment and create a rich foundation for all life activities. While the exercises presented here begin simply, with a focus on the body, their benefits extend to all aspects of our lives. Whatever our interests, occupations, or personal situations, Kum Nye develops our ability to heal and energize the whole of our being. It refreshes the senses and cultivates their higher capacities, opening gateways to experience savored by yogic practitioners of ancient times. Experience accumulates and deepens, unfolding meaning that finds expression in happiness that improves the quality of our actions and our relationships with others. Developing from this foundation, meditation reveals new dimensions of bliss, far beyond what we may now be able to imagine.

This kind of knowledge is missing in modern life, where people tend to equate happiness with having an abundance of money, power, or material possessions, or a prestigious job, or work that one considers important or takes great personal pleasure in pursuing. They may have thought they were living the American Dream by working hard and striving after material goals, only to discover that these goals cannot in themselves produce satisfaction or meaning. Even with hard work, the road to success may be long and beset with problems.

Those who reach their material goals soon find their time filled by job and family responsibilities, by the drive to acquire and maintain possessions, and by a complex array of social and personal obligations. However easy it becomes to possess the latest technology or luxuries unknown to previous generations, many people are not really happy or content.

Shortages are appearing in every area of modern life: shortages of funds, shortages of opportunity, shortages of joy and satisfaction. Day after day, our time is taken over; every moment seems pre-determined, every activity scheduled. Even our entertainments are governed by the pressure of time's constraints. Time seems to be ruling us, squeezing the juice out of every experience.

Simultaneously, distractions abound. Hunger for sensation, or perhaps for escape, leads many to abuse their bodies further by indulging in excesses that complicate their lives still more. However intense these pleasures may be, they tend to be short-lived, and may only increase the driving intensity of desire. At some point we may realize that we are not getting enough enjoyment in life.

Kum Nye awakens joy and helps us make life worth living. Its physical, breathing, massage, and mental exercises promote health of body, mind, and spirit, empowering us to create a positive and productive way of life. We learn how to stimulate the nerves and activate the body centers (cakras) through simple postures and movements. Blockages release and cakras open; vitalizing streams of energy flow through them to and from the senses, supporting the vitality, creativity, and wholeness that expresses the abundance of the human spirit.

By developing the capacities of our senses, we can satisfy the eye hungry for beauty, the mind hungry for meaning, and the heart hungry for love that does not disappoint. We can experience the wealth of pleasures that our senses can provide, so we will never be anxious or lonely, dissatisfied or depressed, yearning and looking for something to fill the emptiness inside. Then it may be possible to manifest the abundance inherent in our nature: abundance of life, abundance of knowledge, and abundance of bliss. If we are inspired to give abundantly as well, we may experience the joy of generosity free from obligation and self-interest. In all these ways, physical, mental, and spiritual, practicing Kum Nye can help us to manifest the bright promise of human being.

The benefits of Kum Nye are fulfilling and convincing; when you experience them for yourself, you will need no further motivation. The yoga of Kum Nye unifies the different aspects of our being and makes us whole. Fully in touch with our own bodies and minds, we can rely on our own resources for happiness. Free of neediness, we can be a good friend to self and others. We will not be so concerned with ordinary problems, but will be sustained with joy in all we do.

Meditation can elevate the yogic practices of Kum Nye into sources of inconceivable bliss so rarified that it goes beyond thought and beyond any sense of self or location in time and place. Since we can become attached to such rapturous experiences, they too will eventually have to be transcended, and accomplishing this will take the guidance of a qualified master. But from where we are now, we need the pleasure that Kum Nye can give to relieve the shortages in our lives and break the patterns that bind us to frustration and pain.

For now, it is important to continue to build and strengthen the Kum Nye experience. These practices stimulate the subtle energies of body and mind. Sensations are likely to become more intense; they may well up spontaneously in ways that enrapture the mind and brighten perceptions, and they may manifest in dreams that communicate deep levels of significance.

If you persist in your practice, you will find that mind and heart have more openness for joy and less and less room for pain and negativity. All these changes are signs that you have begun to embody Kum Nye. From there, you can connect more fully with the spiritual path and follow in the footsteps of the great Bodhisattvas.

2

Our Human Embodiment

The Buddhist tradition teaches that among all possible forms of existence, a human embodiment is the most precious, an opportunity to be treasured and developed as far as our knowledge and circumstances permit. But there is much we do not know about the nature of our embodiment, and until we understand ourselves better, we cannot be truly confident that our knowledge is based on a sound foundation.

Traditional teachings often begin by encouraging students to reflect on how their bodies took form. This can be a valuable exercise that reminds us of how little of our beginnings we actually know and how early the fundamental structures of our bodies and minds were set in place. Since these structures are the basis for the architecture of our being, it is important that we give some thought to how they took form and consider how patterns laid down even before birth may be influencing us today. In the Buddhist tradition, this kind of contemplation fosters understanding of nama-rupa, name-and-form, the founding basis for perception, thought, and action. While not ruling out the wonder and openness of the developing child, the point of this practice is to encourage insight into the patterns of restrictions and pressures that feature in our conditioning and create residues that continue to affect us in our adult lives. If we wish to make positive changes in our lives, examining the roots of our being dispassionately is a good place to begin.

Nama Rupa

We have no direct knowledge of the roots of our being. We have no way to reconstruct the environment in which our bodies took form or appreciate what events and actions may have conditioned that environment.

From what we know now, we can only imagine our development in the womb, with cells dividing and beginning to develop specific functions. For further information, we have to turn to textbooks. We may learn that within weeks, nerve cells start to carry impulses and establish pathways that connect the immature brain to the budding sensory organs. Networks of nerves form in and around the developing senses, defining each organ's future task. If these networks form correctly, the ear will relate to sound, the eye to shapes and forms, and the glands of the nose will respond to odors. Long before food presents itself to the mouth, networks of nerves are beginning to form that will eventually enable the tongue to distinguish tastes and the body to respond to tactile sensations.

It can be awe-inspiring to reflect on the complex interweaving of many hundreds of processes that shape the formation of a human body. What knowledge directs the delicate timing that ensures a good result, and what conditions impede it, however slightly? Already, impulses flowing through the developing brain are stimulating the growth of nerves and setting in place extensive networks for receiving, processing, and feeding back sensory data with electrical speed. Even at this early stage, data carried by the nerves is shaping pathways and interconnecting tissues and organs within the developing embryo.

Physical Birth

We know that sensory development continues after birth, but with a profound change in orientation, as senses open outward for the first time. Even in our imagination, it is difficult to conceive of how profound this change might be, or how we, as infants, may be affected by the tremendous pressures that expel us from our mother's body. The infant cries—reassuring adults that it is taking its first breath, but might it be also a response to the shock of birth?

The infant waves arms and legs; mouth opens and grasps the mother's breast for nourishment; milk streams into the body, calming and satisfying the newborn child. Basic life functions set in motion a multitude of new bodily sensations, and the infant begins to make associations between cries and fulfillment of its needs. The baby's body reacts to heat and cold and to being held and rocked in comforting arms. Sounds, movement, and response establish an elemental form of communication that strengthens through repetition. Simultaneously, the infant's eyes begin to distinguish patterns of light and shadow and the ears hear sounds that may startle and awaken.

Almost from birth, the infant is drawn to stare at the human face, although it will probably be two to four months longer before it recognizes familiar faces. Simultaneously, the faculties for hearing are developing. Among the first sounds the baby may hear is the mother's soft crooning, intended to calm and reassure. Through its body, the infant comes to associate signals with actions, and it expresses hunger and discomfort through cries and physical movements. As experiences accumulate, sounds develop associations with feelings satisfaction, pleasure, discomfort, or fear. With each repetition, sounds, together with their overtones of feelings, become part of the data stream that enters the body, strengthening nerve connections and laying the foundation for later communication.

Shape and Form

As the baby develops, the gates of the senses gradually open, and each organ becomes more sensitive to inner and outer stimulations: The eye interacts with visible forms, the ear with sounds, the nose with smells, the tongue with tastes, the body with forms it can touch and feel, and the mind with mental objects. Raw data pours in through all six of the senses, stimulating nerve synapses and making new connections. But these developing faculties are still immature—how can they sort out what is relevant from this flood of sensory stimulations? What shapes, colors, and textures go with what meaning? What sounds signify what? The foundation is still uncertain, yet from this basis, words develop, words already laden with fragments of associations and connotations.

From amongst these jumbled, overflowing streams of data, points of contact occur; feeling arises, and shape and form are discerned. Someone makes a sound, and the child repeats it. After more repetitions, the child learns the name of the object and can recognize it.

Movement and Restrictions

In the meantime, the child's body is becoming more mobile. Hands can reach out, grasp, and pull. The child learns to turn itself over, to sit up, to crawl about, and finally to stand, around the end of the first year or shortly thereafter. Within a few months or possibly less, the child takes its first steps, and by the end of the next year can also run and climb. With this growth comes awareness of constraints: the child is moved from cradle to crib, strapped in chairs, and set into playpens.

From the time the child begins to move independently, it hears the word "NO!" more and more often, perhaps accompanied by expressions of disapproval and confinement to a safer, and more restricted, place. Restrictions become stronger as the child grows more assertive. Parents begin to direct the child's behavior more energetically, rewarding what they find desirable and restraining or punishing what they find unacceptable. The child may feel frustrated, or act out its feelings in tantrums, upsetting parents and inviting further admonishment or restraint.

Birth of the Self

Although it is not likely that we remember our first efforts to name objects we discern around us, we may observe how the process works, as we see children repeating the sounds that parents make and associating them with an object, more or less accurately. We learn our own names the same way, as if we too were objects. Eventually we learn to say "me." As we begin to string words together, "me" gradually becomes more important, and we say it more and more often. In time, we are able to copy our parents, and say "I." With this, our object-oriented world changes profoundly. "I" am now the subject, assertive and in control. Everything else becomes object, something other than "I."

This transition is not always smooth. It takes a long time before we learn to use the language properly. The concept of "I" is especially difficult, because "I" can also be "me," and objects can also be "mine." With no way to question the use of I, me, and mine, we repeat the patterns the way we hear them from parents or siblings, and by trial and effort eventually get them right. While this switching back and forth subjects us to jokes and laughter, eventually we are able to sort it out. As we copy our parents and older children more accurately, our constant use of I, me, and mine strengthens our sense of self—a self so fundamental and all-encompassing that it soon becomes our basic identity.

Rules and Regulations

Between two and four, we learn the speech and rules of the family. Then we start school and learn new words and different ways of interacting with others. Restraints continue: there are rules we must follow at school and rules to keep us safe. There are rules for language and rules for expressing emotion. There are rules for all manner of social interactions and all kinds of activities.

Childhood unfolds in a context of instructions, admonishments of imminent danger, urgings to "be good," and threats of punishment or deprivation if we are not. At the same time, we are struggling to function outside our family; our sense of self is changeable and insecure. From time to time, we may rebel against rules and restraints that seem to affect everything we do, but ultimately, we have to do as our parents and teachers say; we have to follow the rules.

We go to grade and middle school for eight years, where we are taught more words and concepts; we learn reading and writing, basic arithmetic and science projects, and possibly skills in music and art. Four years in high school follow, with each year growing more complex. We engage in sports and other kinds of activities, each with its own sets of rules and regulations. Our personalities develop, as do new insecurities. We experience conflicts, pressures, and emotional upsets. Nothing seems to fit right—so much we have to do, things we want, things we don't want, things we like or dislike, too many choices, or not enough. We cannot sort through it all, and problems come.

We are now educated, and we graduate. Then, whether or not we feel ready or prepared enough to make sound choices, we have to make decisions that will affect the course of our adult lives. We may take a job or join one of the military services; we may travel for a while, go to college for four to six years, or perhaps longer for a professional degree. At some point, we may marry and start a family. Now we are also occupied with building a career. Along the way we have many desires and distractions; we play games and devise ways to get ahead. We experience blockages; we experiment with alternatives, and we may change course several times.

Now we are in our thirties, or forties, perhaps even fifty or more years of age, and we embody the conditioning that enables us to function in our culture. To a greater or lesser extent, we have accepted the rules and the meanings that have been impressed on us through the years. Whether we have accepted them fully or have tried to shape an independent direction, our behavior has been molded by the expectations of others, and our view of ourselves is likely still to bear the influence of their attitudes and judgments.

Healing with Joy

From where we stand now, we may be able to reflect on what kinds of external experiences have shaped the course of our lives, but we may have no idea how years of restriction have affected the internal aspects of our body: our senses, nerves, organs, and circulatory systems—perhaps even the ways our minds operate. Although our bodies are an ever-present resource for enjoyment and accomplishment, we may have neglected them a long time. Perhaps out of a sense of ownership, we have taken them for granted and abused them with frustration and worries. They may now be suffering from unresolved traumas hidden in the past. They may bear the secret scars of agitation and anger, strong thoughts, and a propensity to rash actions. They may be blocked by knots of tension that close off the flow of feeling.

We now have an opportunity to open these knots from within and bring up the feelings that have been locked within them. Offering the tools we need to relax deeply and open the sensory fields of our being, Kum Nye encourages us to touch sensitive places and embrace strong feelings without fear. Practicing these exercises, we can develop joy that can wash out the painful residues of regret and transform anger and resentment into positive expressions.

As we learn the language of our own bodies and senses, we gain more control over feelings, thoughts, and our style of expression. With an adult consciousness, we can experience freshly the openness of childhood and smooth out the confusion and chaotic associations that seem to be an inevitable outcome of our formative years. We can find our true foundation, improve connections between senses, body and mind, and create a new life for ourselves based on a better understanding of our own embodiment. In a way we have never before experienced, we can truly BE.

3

Tuning In to Relaxation

Certain kinds of sensations, thoughts, and desires that arise during the day tend to create a feeling of discomfort and uncertainty. Although we may not notice their subtle residues, they accumulate as tension in our nerves and muscles, where they constrict the energy of body and mind. We may feel a little down or unhappy, without knowing why or having any idea of how to relieve the feeling. Usually we feel better in the morning when our energy comes up freshly. But the residues have not gone away. They continue to accumulate, and their effects persist, becoming more obvious when our energy slackens.

Most of us realize that we could use a little relaxation when our day's work is done, but we have obligations and responsibilities to fulfill, and it may be difficult to give priority to these needs on a regular basis without feeling somewhat guilty or selfish. In comparison to more strenuous forms of exercise, Kum Nye relaxation may appear very basic and easy, and it is. It makes us feel good, and when we feel good, we can offer positive thoughts and attitudes to others. Relaxation, like other skills, improves with practice, and we get greater benefits if we persevere. Little by little, we get the message, and see for ourselves how greatly Kum Nye can improve the quality of our lives. Although it can take time to realize Kum Nye's full potential, there are pleasant awakenings of interest along the way, and occasional flashes of insight that inspire and delight. We learn how to relieve tension on levels that Western techniques cannot reach, with results that can open doors to the most sublime spiritual experiences.

A Recommended Routine

To create a foundation for practice, establish a regular routine that you can continue daily for several months or more. Prepare for the next day with a light, preferably vegetarian, evening meal, and by relaxing for ten to twenty minutes before going to bed. Upon waking, perform the cleansing exercise.

Cleansing Exercise

Take your seat on a pillow, with legs in the lotus or half-lotus position. If you prefer, the knee of one leg can be raised, with the foot of that leg flat on the floor and facing forward, or you can sit on a chair. Keeping the back straight, with hands palms down on your knees, perform a series of strong exhalations: nine in all, grouped into three sets of three, allowing time to rest in between. Inhale normally, then exhale strongly through both nose and mouth. In each set, do the first two exhalations slowly and the third faster and more heavily. On the final three, exhale as forcibly as you can, as if you were emptying the stomach.

Seated in the same posture, you may vary this exercise as follows: Inhale, then exhale forcefully through both nose and mouth, projecting both arms straight in front of you as you exclaim the syllable, AH! Repeat these movements nine times.

As you perform this exercise, reflect on the residues that are being expelled from your body. You can visualize them as colors carried outward on the breath: dark red, dark black, and a dull muddy color. These residues have feeling tones: dark red carries the feeling tones of anger and revulsion; dark black carries anxiety, grasping, and neediness, and the muddy color carries sluggishness, dullness, and apathy. All these residues—qualities that you feel pressured to express verbally but are emotionally hard to release—can be cleared away on the exhaling breath. With this in mind, exhale strongly and breathe them out completely.

Morning Exercises

Relax the shoulders; move them up and down, then rotate them, one side moving up as the other moves down. Loosen up your chest, and lift it upward a little; move your shoulders a little back to straighten the spine. The back of the neck is straight and aligned with the spine, and the chin is a little tucked in. Stretch the neck by tilting the head, first to one side, so that the right ear moves toward the right shoulder; then tilt to the other side so that the left ear moves toward the left shoulder. Then relax. Repeat these movements nine times, with the neck loosening a little more each time.

If you have no difficulties with your neck, you can include a series of head rotations. You may close your eyes, but keep your mouth open. The breath needs to flow easily through open pathways of both the nose and mouth.

Complete these breathing and movement exercises by relaxing or meditating for fifteen to twenty minutes. Three more times during the day, practice some form of Kum Nye. Posture exercises are particularly good for working into your daily activities. In the evening, before dinner, relax or meditate again for thirty to forty minutes. About an hour or so after dinner, some Kum Nye walking and stretching exercises will help you ease into a good night's sleep. Light but nourishing meals are your best support for practice; rich foods and heavy meals make relaxation more difficult.

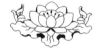

Seven Gestures

The Seven Gestures posture is a balanced way of sitting that allows energy to circulate well through the body. This posture is so effective in promoting relaxation, balance, and integration that it can be used as a complete practice in itself.

1. Select a cushion that is firm and of a comfortable height, thick enough to raise the pelvis above the level of the knees. Sit with your legs crossed, with one leg in front of the other, or, if you prefer, in the half or full lotus. You may also sit with one knee raised and the foot of that leg flat on the floor, or in a straight-backed chair, with both feet flat on the floor and about twelve inches apart. A low meditation bench that allows your legs to be under you will also work well. In all of these variations, the triangle formed by the three points—buttocks and knees—is your essential foundation.

Make yourself comfortable on your seat. Take a few moments to relax and let your limbs ease into place. Experience the sensations in your lower body, such as those where your feet, legs, and pelvis are in contact with the cushion, chair, or bench. In time a sense of being grounded may arise—a firm base for practice.

If you cannot sit on the floor, use a straight-backed chair and sit with both feet on the ground, a comfortable distance apart.

2. With hands on knees (or as far in that direction as they naturally reach), palms down, release tension in the shoul-

ders, and feel the weight of your shoulders and arms as they settle downward. Sense the points of contact between knees or thighs and hands.

3. It is most important that the back is straight and balanced from the base of the spine to the base of the neck so that energy can travel freely from the lower into the upper body. If your back becomes tired, make certain that the top of your pelvis is tilted slightly forward, so that your lower back retains its natural forward curve. Tune in to the sensations in your back and along your spine. Draw the shoulders back a little. Lift the chest slightly and relax tension in the shoulders.

4. Tuck your chin a bit toward your neck, so that the back of the neck is aligned with the spine, and the head balances easily on top of the spinal column without tensing the neck muscles.

5. The mouth is slightly open, with the lips about a half inch apart. This relieves tension in the jaw muscles and allows breath to flow freely, through nose and mouth equally. While it may take a little practice to get accustomed to this way of breathing, it is important to balance the breath by allowing it to flow through both nose and mouth. Breathing through the nose stimulates the head and thoughts, while mouth breathing awakens the body. Breathing through both together helps to gently balance and integrate body and mind, head and heart.

6. The tip of the tongue is lightly touching the ridge of the palate, just behind the front teeth. The tip of the tongue is slightly curled back, and the tongue is relaxed.

7. The eyes are open with a soft, panoramic gaze. Notice muscle tension around the eyes and let it melt away.

You can minimize the need to blink by relaxing the area around your eyes and drawing your awareness inward. This happens naturally when you soften the focus of your eyes and imagine you are looking inward, toward the back of the eyeballs.

It can take several weeks for your body to relax fully into this position. It is important to remind yourself that with practice, small discomforts will soon ease, allowing you to sit comfortably for longer periods of time. It is not necessary to struggle to create a sense of stability. If you start with the body comfortable and the back straight, your body will develop its own points of balance. You may sense small shifts from time to time; this is perfectly normal, and you can enjoy the subtle feelings that often accompany these shifts.

Listen to your body for guidance on how to explore experience in a new way, not necessarily with words, but in movement. Each sensation or feeling or sound or thought is its own gesture, and each of these feeling-gestures can be the seed of fresh experience.

Within each gesture there is a movement that makes it more expressive or eloquent. This movement also moves you and awakens you. As you are being moved, joy may arise, or perhaps clarity. Every movement and every moment can be meaningful.

Some of these gestures can be practiced separately at any time during the day, such as the placement of the tongue, the nose-and-mouth breathing, the balancing and straightening of the back together with releasing the shoulder tension.

This practice is beneficial from the outset. While the initial release of tension it promotes may be refreshing, ecstatically joyful, or even evoke tears of relief, it is important to remember that sustained practice will lead to far greater benefits. Participating in retreats, twice a year if possible, will give even more satisfying results.

After about forty-eight hours of practice, you may begin to notice feelings in a new way. As you listen to their rhythms and follow their momentum, you may sense them as tones that resonate in the body with an almost musical quality, leading to a deeper and more blissful sense of relaxation. Let yourself merge with the feelings that arise; ease yourself into them and allow them to expand.

Creating a New Home of Feeling

Developed in this way, feelings that arise from deep relaxation transform our physical environment into a warm, comfortable home. Consciousness becomes brighter and more positive, open to new ideas and change. Fresh surges of vigor and vitality inspire an inner remodeling of our way of being. Expanded and deepened, this practice reveals the beauty of our own spiritual qualities and leads naturally into meditation. Once we have created this home, we can enter it whenever we wish.

As you continue your practice, you may find the sense of ease and relaxation extends into more and more of your daily activities. Familiar patterns tend to repeat themselves, memories come up, bringing with them fantasies and other kinds of imaginings and reverie, but all of this mental activity can become part of your relaxation process. However attractive they may be, or however you might wish to push them away, pay them no attention—just let them be. Relax your body, stay with the sense of ease and relaxation, and let go all the manifestations of mental activity. As they fade, sink more deeply into your inner home of relaxation, and allow them to completely drop away.

If emotions and inner dialogues continue to interfere, take this opportunity to practice melting them into calmness. Breathing through nose and mouth, relax deeply; without responding to the stories spinning through the mind, listen to the flow of sound and let your mental chatter fade into meaningless sounds and rhythms. As the energy of high pitched, demanding thoughts calms down, you can deepen relaxation and surrender completely to peace and tranquility.

Regular practice will develop your ability to melt into calmness in this way, so encourage yourself to relax as fully as possible at least twice a day. Once you have tasted the feeling of relaxation, it is important to understand that thoughts have no substance in themselves. When they come up, remind yourself that there is no need to avoid them, restrain them, or push them away.

Relaxation can accommodate whatever arises in the mind; relaxation can smooth the jagged edges of thoughts, remove their hooks from our consciousness, and enable them to slip away. Experience gives us the confidence we need to make room even for uncomfortable thoughts and upsetting emotions. Eventually, if we continue to persevere in our practice, Kum Nye can empower us to embrace all negative thoughts and emotions and transform them into compassion. The healing energy of compassion relieves remnants of guilt and self-doubts that may now lie too deep for expression. As we develop Kum Nye further, we can use it even more effectively, in ways that reveal themselves naturally over time.

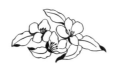

4

Tuning Up and Tuning In

How often do we want to accomplish something, but feel blocked by a sense of restraint that we do not fully understand? Perhaps there is something we want to express, but cannot find the right words. There are plenty of reasons—"I don't know how," "No one has taught me that," "I don't want to make a mistake," "I can't do it." But reasons do not help us accomplish our purpose, and even we may realize that such reasons are not really reasons at all—they have no solid ground. Often we have no idea of why the resistance is there, so we cannot dissolve it by thinking it through. Caught between the need or desire to do and the reasons why we cannot, we become tense—tied up in knots—that we have no way to release. We put off, delay, and procrastinate, and in doing so miss valuable opportunities that set us up for regret.

Just Do It Now!

When you are stressed and in serious need of relief, the thought may come, "I don't know how to do it—I don't know how to relax." The only way you can do it is to feel out points of tenseness in the body and relax them one by one, as much and as often as possible. At various times during the day, or as part of your regular seated practice, wherever you sense a tight, holding quality, release it. Let go of demanding thoughts—the "I don't know how" that is constricting your mind. Let go of the "I" that is identifying you with confusion. All these thoughts are irrelevant—confusion is irrelevant, reasons are irrelevant, and fixating on "I" is not helpful. At these times you only know you are tense and uncomfortable.

So loosen up all parts of the body: relax the nerves in the chest, and just let be. Relax your throat, letting the jaw drop open slightly. Half-close your eyes and soften your gaze. Gently stretch the back of your neck slightly, and relax the muscles there. Scan your body again for signs of tenseness. Wherever you notice tightness or tension, release it. Breathe softly, and rest the mind in calmness.

In practicing Kum Nye, your best friend is patience—patience with yourself, based on the knowledge that you deserve a relaxed, healthy body and mind, and developing them is well worth the effort. It usually takes several weeks to catch on to how to work with tensions and body sensations to the point where you begin to sustain a calm and steady state of relaxation. This initial stage prepares you for the process of "tuning up" the body, mind, and senses, calming them and orienting them to a relaxed state of being that is quiet, completely open, and free of fixations. This process is similar to tuning up the engine of a car to make it run more smoothly, energetically, and efficiently.

With sustained practice, as you progress to a more advanced level, you will be able to embrace whatever thoughts and feelings pop up by melting their energy into the calmness of relaxation. Eventually, there will be nothing left that is not relaxed.

These instructions are merely suggestions as to ways to proceed. As you work with these techniques, you may find yourself creating your own recipe for noting and releasing tension. Since Kum Nye tends to inspire innovation, you are encouraged to follow the flow of feeling and your own bodily responses.

Easing Pain and Emotionality

However much we have cared for the exterior appearance of our bodies, we have not understood their inner mechanisms well, and so have taken them largely for granted. While our bodies have been shaped by restrictions and rules imposed by social conditioning and education, our minds and senses have largely developed on their own, absorbing the consequences of our attitudes and behavior, but without much awareness or conscious guidance on our part. As a result, they are now tuned in to negativity: more sensitive to pain than to pleasure, more easily attracted to catastrophe than to contentment, more confident with negativity than with positive attitudes, more readily magnetized to problems than inspired to creative thought and action.

The focus of the mind and senses are now oriented to events outside the body; responsive to external stimulation, they tend to rely more strongly on external than internal sources for meaning and satisfaction. In a sense, we might say they have abandoned us, looking outside in search of nourishment we have not been able to provide, leaving us dependent on objects and events outside our control.

It is important to attract mind and senses back to their natural home, where we can tune in to our own inner resources for meaning and satisfaction. We need to connect heart and head, so their energies can cooperate and flow freely, unifying soul, spirit, and self into a new sense of being.

We can invite calmness and joyful feelings to circulate throughout our systems, healing emotional distress and easing physical pain. Although more advanced practices are necessary to transform intense pain and emotions completely, by working with the following exercise, we can begin to protect ourselves from their harmful effects.

When intense pain or strong emotions come up, try to make a gap, so the sharpness of the feeling does not hit you directly. You might visualize pain as if it were a wave of aliens coming toward you, fierce beings you can hold off by the power of awareness. Feel awareness radiating from you like a forcefield that the pain-aliens can touch, but not penetrate. Use awareness to hold the sharp emotion or pain at a distance. It may come so close that you can feel its vibrations right against you, but do not let it come in.

If you can extend this forcefield, if you can open a gap between yourself and the pain, it will not hit you directly, and you can escape the full force of its sharpness. If you do not know how to make that gap, use your memory to recall beautiful experiences, bring them to the present, intensify them, and focus on opening a tiny space between you and the pain. Then you can allow energy to expand that space further so it can serve as your protection.

With sustained practice, Kum Nye develops the ability to open this space and provides a reservoir of energy that can empower awareness even more. From that foundation, oral instructions from a qualified master are necessary to reveal more profound levels of significance inherent in this practice.

Remembering Joy

The powerful feelings awakened through the practice of Kum Nye can flood our being with relief and joy, as if we had been searching for a long time and had finally come home after a long and difficult journey. Once this intensity of feeling touches the heart, we may be able to extend the current of feeling further and keep it alive in memory, from where we can recall it at will. Then the fresh joy of experience will not just come about by accident, but will be available as a constant source of spiritual strength and renewal. This is a therapeutic practice that you can apply whenever you wish.

This deep current of feeling carries with it the sweetness of intimacy and the radiant glow of love. When we keep it alive in heart and mind, experience becomes an ongoing celebration, a love affair with our own spiritual path. The intensity of feeling transforms our being: the quality of our embodiment is noticeably different and relationships—to the senses, to thoughts, to the people we care for—may also be greatly improved.

While this path may sound somewhat selfish, and may look different from the way of the Bodhisattva, it enables us to rely on ourselves—to find our own home and develop our own resources, to become friends with our own mind, body, and senses.

If you continue to develop your practice, you may someday be inspired to share it with others and encourage them through your example. If you would like to emulate the example of the great Bodhisattvas, you can begin by dedicating the merit of your practice to all sentient beings, wishing that they might also have this experience.

How to Nurture Compassion

Once upon a time, an Indian king asked the Buddha, "What are the most meritorious actions I can possibly do? Can you give me any instructions?" In reply, Buddha advised him to wish all sentient beings well, and to dedicate to them all meritorious actions done by anyone in the past. Following the Buddha's advice, we too can dedicate whatever positive thoughts and feelings we have accumulated to the benefit of others. This is a simple yet important practice that leads to the growth of wisdom and compassion.

Until our understanding is grounded in experience, our words and gestures are not truly our own, and they cannot carry much merit. However well-intentioned our wishes may be, however much we feel they come from the bottom of the heart, if we lack the experience to know what such phrases mean, they may be little more than social conventions. But once we have knowledge, we may find we also have a new way to communicate. Our words come from a more wholesome place and are more true to our being. The deeper and more meaningful our experience, the more merit our wishes and prayers can convey, and the more they will benefit others.

Someday practitioners in the West may understand more fully what the Bodhisattvas' gestures of compassion signify. What is the meaning of their tears and their smiles? Do their tears indicate that they see us trapped in samsara and wish to liberate us from our confusion? Do they smile to uplift us with their blessings?

To comprehend the full significance of these gestures, we need to experience for ourselves what it means to be a genuinely selfless being, free of doubts and uncertainties instilled by our conditioning, and endowed with boundless compassion for all sentient life. When we too can see with the eyes of enlightened compassion, our words and gestures will be truly sincere, beneficial to all beings in all ways.

5

Embodying Kum Nye

To embody means to give form to a quality or an idea, to manifest something intangible so we can relate to it in a more tangible way. In that sense, we might say, to embody Kum Nye is to manifest the quality of being—a vibrant aliveness fully attuned to the present moment. Being makes possible the rich array of feelings that give pleasure and meaning to human life. While we tend to associate being most closely with the body, being is the property of a fully integrated whole that encompasses body, senses, and mind—in other words, a complete human being.

When we practice Kum Nye, our initial focus is on relaxing the body, using massage, postures, and movement to release deeply-held tensions and stimulate the circulation of vital energies through our entire body system. As described in *Kum Nye Tibetan Yoga* and presented in the last section in this book, these practices promote health and well-being, while calming the restless tendencies of body and mind that interfere with the development of meditation. On a more advanced level, learning to stay with the flow of feeling relaxes and refreshes the senses as well, and opens their capacities for greatly enriching the quality of our lives.

When we move more deeply into these practices, we learn that they can awaken intensities of feeling that fill our consciousness with light and bring beauty and joy into our lives as an ongoing celebration. Along the way, we may have some glimpses into how embodying Kum Nye benefits the mind. These glimpses remind us that, while theory can point the way, only direct experience makes knowledge truly our own. This is the knowledge that empowers growth and change and comes alive in every gesture of our being.

Touching the Essence of Feeling

Kum Nye relaxes the body, calming the mind and slowing down the speed of perceptions and thoughts. Gradually, usually after several weeks of daily practice, the mind settles more readily into a quiet attentiveness, alert, but not grasping for thoughts or fixating on perceptions. With body relaxed and mind more cooperative, we can attune our senses to a greater intensity of feeling. Just as powerful engines propel a rocket into space, and then drop away when their purpose is accomplished, our senses can generate blissful feelings, then release, allowing the mind to enter the deep calm of meditation.

Make yourself comfortable in the Seven Gestures posture and breathe through both nose and mouth. With the back of the neck straight, aligned with the spine, relax neck and shoulders. Lift the chest slightly and allow the arms to fully relax. Sense any remaining areas of tension, and relax them with the breath.

When feeling arises, relax into the sensation, but do not go into it in a grasping way, seeking for meaning. As much as possible, stay with the pure flavor of the feeling, without losing yourself in thoughts or emotionality. Savor the feeling deeply and allow it to expand. With practice, the feeling will intensify, becoming almost tangible. Sustained practice will purify the flavor of the feeling; eventually only the essence will remain.

Benefits of Cultivating Rich Depths of Feeling

When we cultivate our capacity for experiencing rich depths of feeling, life becomes an ongoing symphony of feelings that blend and harmonize throughout the day, sustaining us with interest, creativity, and positive thoughts. Discords come, but they also resolve and merge into the inherently joyous and uplifting momentum of life's unfolding. The more attuned we become to the positive aspects of experience, the more good feelings accumulate in body and mind, and the more completely we embody them. Gradually we build up reserves of joy that invite the blessings of bliss into our practice. Bliss cannot be bought with material riches or given us by others, but we can invite it and allow it to develop. Once established, bliss becomes our property, our own creation, and it shines through every action of our body, speech, and mind. When hard times come, we can draw upon these blessings to restore our balance and reach out to others with love and appreciation.

However inspiring it may be to theorize about what is possible, teachings without practice may only distance us further from the vitality of direct experience. So it is important to take encouragement from the examples of the Arhats and great siddhas, who knew how to use the energy of body, mind, and senses to realize profound states of bliss. If we too have access to these treasures, we owe it to ourselves to develop them, and Kum Nye gives us a way. So we need not be shy about getting inside our experience and embracing it intimately, below the level of concepts. Viewing our own embodiment as a precious resource, we may find our joy.

We have been on a long journey; the road has been long and difficult at times, and it is time to make it better. We can heal our senses and transform them into our best friends and constant companions; we can reclaim the joy and peace that is our human heritage and become examples for others who are lonely and isolated, vulnerable to frustration and pain. If even a few practitioners can demonstrate how to develop the capacities of their mind, body, and senses, others will be inspired to join them, adding their energy to illumine for us all the journey to a richer and fuller way of being.

Part Two

Breath

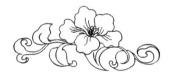

The three pillars of spiritual practice are relaxation, meditation, and concentration. Each pillar has skillful methods for transforming the quality of our lives, energizing body and mind, dissolving obstacles to understanding, and awakening the full capacities of human being. Anyone who wishes to focus on Kum Nye can benefit from the inner and outer massage of its postures and movements.

Kum Nye can be practiced as a way to relieve tension and agitation; it can be used to sharpen sensory perceptions and bring more beauty and joy into our lives; it can be used to calm body and mind and ease us gently into meditation, and it can become a gateway to sublime states of bliss.

The foundation for receiving all of these benefits is our own embodiment: our physical systems, traditionally known as nadi, and our vital energies, or vayu, beginning with the breath.

6

Breath, Energy, Feeling

Kum Nye is based on comprehensive understanding of the body: how its inner systems operate, how
they are interconnected, and how they are activated by
energy (vayu) circulating through them. Five distinct kinds
of energy condition the overall environment of the body.
Some circulate in muscle, blood vessels, nerves, and other
types of tissues; some are specific to the six sensory organs,
and others sustain the functions of our digestive, renal,
and autonomic systems. The primary vayu is the energy
of breath, which stimulates all of the vital organs, including liver, heart, lungs, and kidneys, and supports our entire
physical system. Exercises based on mindfulness of breath
can improve circulation of energy throughout the body and
promote the health of our vital organs.

Masters of yoga know how energy flows throughout the
body; like skilled travelers directing their mounts through
complex terrain, they can direct the movement of their

energy properly to accomplish their spiritual practices. Although we are not at this level, we can make good use of this knowledge to relax body, mind, and senses.

Basic Mindfulness of Breath

When the body relaxes, breath responds by flowing more smoothly, entering and leaving the body in a regular, even rhythm. Wherever you are and whatever you are doing, you can observe this flow of breath, feeling the quality of the breath as it moves through the nostrils and into the lungs. Notice if the breath is shallow or deep, how deeply it moves into the chest, and the way the diaphragm is moving to accommodate the flow of air. Sense or visualize the breath passing through the membranes of the lungs into the arteries, and follow the movement of energy throughout the body, as it flows into the vital organs and cakras and stimulates nerves, glands, and muscles.

When energy flows smoothly through the body, through the vital organs and cakras, you feel energized and alert; the mind is clear, nerves are poised for transmitting signals, and muscles are ready for movement. The mind also responds and becomes more tranquil and cooperative. As thoughts become less impulsive and demanding, you can sustain focus and concentration and direct your energy in a more open, relaxed manner.

Observing the movement of breath while inhaling and exhaling, you may notice a kind of flavor, a sense of calm that grows stronger as you continue. Gradually, this sensation becomes fuller and deeper, developing into calmness that you can broaden and intensify. The senses become more fully alive, producing deep tones of feeling that resonate through the body centers, releasing feelings that soothe and calm the nerves. Body and mind relax further, as the flow of feeling intensifies and spreads, nurturing the entire being on a deeper, more organic level. As much as possible, deepen and stabilize this flow of feeling. As you rest in this calmness, any stimulus you experience can produce very pleasurable sensations, nourishing the mind and turning it toward bliss.

In breathing out, your breath connects the energy of body to energies outside, linking it to the positive energies of the environment, space, and the cosmos. Breathing in, you invite these energies inside, encouraging a subtle communication of inner and outer that stimulates and revitalizes body and mind. The feeling tone produced can become very joyful, even ecstatic. Advanced yogic practitioners are said to be able to bring the essence of the five elements into the cakras through their meditation. So effectively can they nourish themselves with cosmic energy that they can live on very little physical food.

Even on the common level, our inner and outer environments seem to be closely related. Energy in the environment communicates with our inner energy, and each may affect how we view the other. For example, a bright sunny day with clean, fresh air calls forth a bright and positive outlook, while overcast skies and closed rooms with damp, stale air make us more vulnerable to dullness and depression. Some types of people are especially sensitive as to how the environment and other external situations affect their bodies, feelings, and thoughts, while others would deny that such synergy exists. But whether we recognize it or not, our bodies respond to external energy as well as internal.

Awakening Feeling

Where, then, are the seeds or the roots of our energy? The way to this knowledge is through relaxation. Sit quietly, and allow mind to relax deeply, as if you were looking into a deep pool, pure as crystal and blue as the open sky. See the pool as very still and calm; invite this deep calming quality into your body. Breathe it in, and allow it to pass through the throat and into the lungs; feel it warming the heart and relaxing the abdomen. When sounds come, listen for the stillness that continues on, as sound itself comes and goes. Allow mind and body to enter that stillness, following it as it deepens and expands. When feeling arises, surrender to it, relaxing completely. Let go of words, let go of concepts, let go of interpretations, and simply be one with whatever feeling comes. Melt into the feeling, taste the calmness, and relish the stillness enveloping mind and body. Sounds come and go; thoughts may drift through the mind like clouds through the sky, but the calmness remains. Rest in that tranquil, yet dynamic space, open to communication from within and without. Begin by practicing this exercise for fifteen minutes and gradually extend the time to sessions of thirty to forty minutes.

Energizing Flow of Feeling

Energy flows into the heart cakra, and from there circulates to all parts of the body. As you breathe in through nose and mouth, with jaw loose and relaxed, feel the breath touching and opening the throat, relaxing any areas of tension in the throat and neck. When the throat feels relaxed, allow the breath to touch the heart, comforting it with warmth.

The heart deserves our care and compassion. It is a universal symbol of love, yet how often do we remember to replenish it by offering it our love? It beats faithfully for us hour after hour, day after day, sharing our joys and suffering our sorrows through good times and bad, always doing their best to fulfill our demands.

When you do this exercise, turn your thoughts to your heart and use this opportunity to offer it love and appreciation. Sense the feelings as they ebb and flow with the breath, touching the heart like a gentle massage. Relax deeply into the feelings; let them completely envelop you with gentle warmth. The sense of aliveness awakened through relaxation flows through the cakras, sense organs, and the body systems, radiating outside as well as inside the body. As you practice, you may sense the body becoming lighter, as if it were touching space or extending into space, beyond the physical form.

Connecting Inner and Outer

As you develop the sense of connection between inner and outer, between the calmness within and the openness of space around your body, you can invite more of the fresh open quality of space into your cakras and inner tissues and enjoy a deeper level of relaxation. Touching space in this way cultivates a sense of the body floating in space, profoundly calm, yet vibrant with a deep silent joy. This exercise is an excellent way to relax tension and prepare mind and body for a sound, refreshing night's sleep.

Continue to develop this practice in daily sessions of forty-five minutes. In time, the feeling of lightness becomes part of you, merged with the tissues of your body. Thoughts also become lighter and inner dialogues less distracting. Eventually thoughts will melt more readily into space. Feelings of joy and peace will also lighten, as the body relaxes further into the openness of space. As body sensations drop away, at some point thoughts and feelings may become so light and open they may seem to have evaporated into thin air. When body and mind are totally open, there remains only the sense of spaciousness, in which you may glimpse the quality that some masters have called the lightness of being. When you mature in this practice, you can enter this field of being whenever you wish.

7

Attuning Body and Breath

Body and breath are the foundation of our being, the basis for relaxation and meditation. Together, they serve as our meditation cushion, the support for our practice and also for our lives. The better they function, the more stable will be our practice and the more certain our development. So it is important to make the body comfortable and allow the breath to become gentle and relaxed. Then we can work with Kum Nye.

Calming Body and Breath

Various exercises may recommend different positions, the most usual being the lotus or half-lotus positions, or the half-lotus with one knee raised and the foot flat on the floor in front of the body. A chair or a meditation bench may also be used. In all of these positions, it is important to sit in a balanced way, with a firm foundation and a straight spine.

The back of the neck is aligned with the spine, and the head is well-balanced on the body so that there is no strain on the neck, and the neck muscles are relaxed. The chin is a little back and slightly lowered, roughly aligned with the larynx. The eyes are half open, relaxed and soft, not blinking. The tip of the tongue can be slightly curled and raised toward the upper palate, but not necessarily touching it. If you sense tension, let the tongue rest a little lower. The mouth is open, with the lips a little apart, allowing room for the breath to flow in and out of the mouth. The hands rest on or near the knees, palms down. (For a more detailed description, see the Seven Gestures, page 21.)

Take a few minutes to loosen up the body, letting tension drain away. Let your breath slow and ease into a gentle rhythm. Exhale gently, and inhale through the nose and the mouth, allowing the breath to come in very softly. Breathing may become so light and gentle that you may not even notice it flowing in and out.

During the rest of the day, when you relax or meditate in the seven gestures position, continue to keep the mouth open and breathe through both nose and mouth. Breathing through the mouth is an esoteric technique that helps practitioners settle more easily into meditation. Although other meditation traditions may tell you to close the mouth, it is important that you become accustomed to keeping the mouth slightly open and breathing through both nose and mouth. The nostrils are sensitive and closely connected with the mind and nervous system. Breathing through the nose stimulates thoughts and emotions, activating the perceptual process, but most practitioners do not understand how this works or realize how easily their own thoughts can deceive them. They may feel they are getting somewhere, while actually there may be little progress.

Tuning the Breath

Breath is our vital energy, the engine that powers our being. All our actions depend on the quality of our breath and the way it circulates in the body. The ability to calm and regulate the breath enables us to control emotions and thought; we call this process "tuning the breath." As yoga practitioners have demonstrated, breath can be used to quiet mental activity completely and transform it into bliss. The Ayurvedic traditions associate breath with longevity, noting that there have been yogic sages in the past who have lived a very long time, using breath as only source of nourishment.

Allow the breath to become as light as possible, with the breath coming in and out in a way that is hardly noticeable. The chest feels comfortable, and the body relaxes. After two or three weeks, you may observe that the breath flowing in is a light sky-blue color, with a gentle feeling-tone that flows inside and heals the body. When you exhale, feel all the tension while it is being released, passing completely out of the body. As the breath comes back, it fills body and senses with the healing nectar of relaxation.

If you do not see the blueness of the breath, you can visualize the breath coming into and passing out of your body. Even as the breath moves in and out, it is never actually gone. As long as you live, your body has an abundance of this healing nourishment that supports a continual flow of energy through your senses, muscles, and organs. Inhale, sensing this stimulation; exhale gently, breathing out tension and letting it go. Do this twenty-five times each session, feeling the rhythm of the breathing, with just a little attention to counting.

As you develop this practice and become more attuned to the rhythms of your breathing, you will relax further, and the breath will be smoother and slower. The breath can become so slow and light that you may hardly notice it at all, perhaps as slow as one minute for each complete cycle of inhaling and exhaling. At first, inhalation and exhalation have distinct high and low points, but as the breath slows and calms, these points smooth out more and more, until there is no interruption in the rhythm, and in and out merge into a single smooth cycle.

Practice tuning the breath for two hours a day for two to three weeks to develop the experience of calming and relaxation. Remind yourself to inhale and exhale through nose and mouth equally, letting the breath come and go, modulating it with just a little control, yet loose enough to quiet the impulsiveness of mind and senses. Be sensitive to the flow of breath; as this exercise develops, you will be increasingly able to relax the senses and thoughts.

If possible, develop this practice further during the course of a two to four week retreat. Practice tuning the breath to a gentle, calm rhythm four to five hours during the day. Allow the breath to soften and become very calm and slow. Within the breath, you may sense a quality of stillness; as your practice develops, this stillness becomes more noticeable as sweet, even joyful feelings of calm and peace. When that stage is fully established, tension dissipates, and the breath can be controlled without conscious effort. Breathing in and out becomes so smooth that you may not even notice you are breathing, and breathing itself becomes like space.

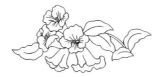

8

Being Present through Breath

*F*rom time to time during the day, pay attention to the breath. Practice observing the rhythms and pace of your inhalations and exhalations. If you feel emotional or anxious, allow the breath to slow down and go more deeply into the lower part of the chest. Allow the muscles of the lower abdomen to relax and come forward, making room for the breath to move lower into the body. Note what feelings arise; breathe into the feelings, and take note of how breath connects with feeling.

Short Breath

Begin by relaxing, as described earlier in Calming Body and Breath. Notice the flow and intensity of the breath as you inhale and exhale, and allow the movements to soften and fall into a natural rhythm. Listen attentively to the breath entering the lungs and circulating through all parts of the body. Feel the expanding and condensing as breath moves into the chest, signals the diaphragm to relax, and flows into the lower abdomen. Sense the breath touching and flowing into your inner organs, and feel the rhythmic expanding and condensing of your breath massaging them, stimulating a flow of feeling that warms and revitalizes. Sink into these feelings, taste their sweetness, and listen for their tones, even if they manifest as silence. After several weeks or so, you may notice changes in the quality of this silence and the feelings that come as you listen. Savor the calmness that these feelings evoke; encourage it to deepen and expand by relaxing further and breathing into the feelings.

Practice this exercise for fifteen to twenty minutes, two times a day.

Long Breath

Sensory impulses have flavors, not flavors that we can readily identify in words, but subtle flavors we might associate with such qualities as sweetness, warmth, melting, or glowing. When we listen to music, for example, we recognize notes, melodies, rhythm, and specific voices and instruments. But within these readily identifiable elements, there are undertones and qualities of fullness and depth. When we contemplate the breath, these and other elements can be brought in to "season" our meditation, to stimulate it and make it richer. To experience how this works, you can reflect on very pleasant memories. Gently massage these memories with your breath as you breathe in and out, allowing pleasurable feelings to come up and spread through your body. Focusing gently on these sensations, let specific meanings and associations fall away, until only the quality of the feeling remains—sweetness, perhaps, or vibrant clarity. No object, no associations, only the inner essence of the feeling continues. This feeling-essence merges with your meditation, stimulating and energizing it.

Follow the energy as it flows like a deep inner shower under and over tissues, into the organs and cells, warming all parts of the body, sustaining your life, and stimulating the joy of being alive. Feel this energy touching and activating the senses; merge it with sensations, feeling-tones, and memories. Whatever thoughts or feelings this practice stirs up, let them merge into the breath. Breathe them out as you exhale, and bring them in as you inhale. Taste the feelings that wash over you; relish them and let them carry you along. Mind and senses are alert, filled with feelings of deep joy. At the same time, there is stillness and meditation, a sense of continuity and connection of inner and outer. You are complete; you are perfect, just as you are.

Practice this longer exercise for forty minutes, twice each day. This is the first stage. When you can taste and enjoy the flavor of experience, when you feel good about yourself and comfortable in your body, you can see for yourself the treasures that can be cultivated. This is the way to enrich the ground of meditation and prepare the foundation for enlightenment.

Deepening through Breath

The longer you can extend the feeling of this stimulation, the more sensitive you become to the flow of energy produced. If you focus on the throat cakra, you can sense the flow of energy as it moves to the heart and navel and disperses throughout the nerves and muscles. In every place it touches, especially the sensitive areas of the body, you may feel soft warmth, a melting, buttery sensation that relaxes and heals. As you relish the flavor of this experience, the mind attunes itself to the senses and communicates pleasurable thoughts that intensify the feelings still more: "How wonderful it is to be so completely in touch with my body and feelings—so completely whole! How refreshing it is to just be still in this way!"

If you wish, you can focus on the cakras, concentrating on one after the other, or, if you prefer, on another part of the body, or even outside it. The breath goes to all cells of the body; it does not stop with the skin, but passes in and out through the cells of the skin as well. Continue to follow the breath as it passes through the skin and out into space as you exhale, then comes back into the body as you inhale. Feel the tissues of the muscles and inner organs relax more with each breath, allowing more space to open, until the spaces between the cells become clear pathways for air and light. Allow light to flow in and illumine the cells of the muscles, the heart, the lungs, and the lower belly, then follow it as it flows out again, shining in space.

Sense this light merging with your vital energy, awakening intensely joyful feelings. Join these feelings too with the flow of breath, drawing them into your body with each inhalation. As your breath pauses before changing direction, allow the feelings to intensify, then intensify the feelings further as you exhale. Even the space outside your body relaxes. Your entire body becomes translucent and light, like a crystal bowl filled with milk and water, full of the flavor of feeling.

You may remember wonderfully happy times from your childhood. As you meditate with the breath, you can use your memory to bring them in to the present. Whatever good thoughts or imagery come up, add them like seasonings to your meditation to release the full juiciness of the feelings. The whole experience becomes sweet like nectar, melting all pockets of tension, smoothing and energizing all parts of the body. The senses come fully alive, adding their distinctive tones to the nectar of feeling. You can taste it and touch it. You can attune your ears to its silent melodies and fill your consciousness with bliss. When bliss fills body and mind, rest within it: there is no tension, no thoughts, no concepts—there is only bliss. Nothing else is needed, there is nothing else you need to do.

When you are just beginning to learn how to swim, as soon as you feel comfortable in the water, you can enjoy the feeling of floating or gentle movement without thinking about how to do it. Similarly, when you know how to get inside the feelings Kum Nye awakens, you can carry on the flavor of that experience without thinking about instructions. Eventually, as you walk or go about your work, your Kum Nye experience will remain steady, following along with you without paling out. While you are engrossed in physical work or in making decisions, you could also be doing these breathing exercises, for both of these activities have similar flavors in the all-embracing field of awareness.

Meditators of all traditions can benefit from the physical health and mental balance developed through this practice. When we taste the bliss possible through this practice, meditation becomes easy.

Engaging the Field of Perception

As we develop the ability to relax deeply, our energy becomes gentle, almost tender, flowing more freely into the senses and bathing them in rich, flavorful experiences. Thoughts are attracted to share in the joy; they connect more completely with perceptions, lending their powers to open new fields of perception. Objects we see have deeper significance that nourishes us with meaning; sounds we hear resonate in our bodies and merge with our own inner rhythms; fragrances focus and still the mind more effectively, and tastes give more pleasure.

The more we enter into this wider and deeper field of perception, the more we dwell in awareness of abundance that is truly our own. We embody more of the fullness of experience, more of the dynamic momentum of life itself. The flavor of experience can become celestial ambrosia, the source of joy that transports mind to the heavenly realms.

Knowledge gained from this practice can become our armament for the spiritual path, and awareness, sustained by our field of perceptions, can protect us from losing our way.

A Path of Transformation

Western students may find it difficult to relate to traditional religious ceremonies, or they may lack the depth of faith and devotion needed to benefit quickly from traditional forms of practice. For them, as well as for those following a traditional approach, Kum Nye offers a path to transformation that does not depend on specific sadhanas or difficult yogic practices. Following the example of the great Arhats, we can use the body, mind, and senses as the foundations of our practice.

Through Kum Nye, we can use our ordinary senses and perceptions to tune into profound and expansive states of mind and achieve faster results. Wherever mind, senses and consciousness operate, we can get the flavor of experience, feel it deeply, and allow it to become one with the alert calmness of meditation. If we develop the properties of our own embodied being, we can ultimately arrive at the same sublime states as highly developed yogic masters and Bodhisattvas.

Part Three

Senses and Perception

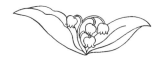

The great Bodhisattvas unite karuna, enlightened compassion, with upaya, the skillful means that transform all substances and actions into a smooth and pleasant path. Although we are not at this level of spiritual understanding, we can use Kum Nye to experience beautiful thoughts and feelings.

Day and night, in crowds or alone, we can use our senses to practice distilling the pure juice of all perceptions and experiences, and allowing all the dross to drop away. When we learn how this works, Kum Nye can truly make our day.

Through relaxation, all manner of mental and physical experience can be turned into a positive flow of energy that stimulates good feelings and abundant vitality. The experience of beauty, for example, can awaken thoughts and feelings laid down earlier in life and bring them into the present in a very powerful way. The experience of faith can connect with thoughts that magnify the experience and awaken a new dimension of spiritual sensitivity.

Long-hidden treasures of mind begin to manifest, emerging like beautiful jewels from the depths of a clear pool. Kum Nye enables us to connect with these jewels, bring them into the light, and share them with others.

9

Generating Happiness
from Within

*E*veryone wants happiness, but few know how to generate it independently from within. Our bodies, minds,
and sense organs are the source of our vital energies, but
all too often these energies are directed into pain, com-
plaints, and dissatisfaction that work from within to close
our hearts and isolate us from others. We have only to look
around us to see where this negative current leads. Can seeing this inspire us to develop a more positive orientation?
Can we ask mind and senses to give us more pleasure and
less pressure? Can we ask ourselves for contentment and
inner peace, the foundation for satisfaction and joy that
does not depend upon others?

Since the time of the Buddha, great Arhats and yogic
masters have known how to enter the most sublime states of
peace and joy at will, and have been able to sustain themselves there in perfect equanimity. While devotion, prayer,

and meditation can give access to profoundly blissful and transformative experiences, few individuals have the background and training to engage them directly. Today we may benefit more quickly from Kum Nye relaxation techniques that develop the capacities of the senses and enable us to accommodate deep levels of meditation.

Kum Nye relieves the tension that closed the senses and deprived the mind of calmness and satisfaction. It opens the senses more widely to beauty and joy and restores our inner light, enabling us to get the juice of all kinds of experience. As our practice develops, our perceptions may provide us with very pleasant surprises. Sounds, sights, smells, colors, objects, memories, positive feelings, and wishes, even negative thoughts and emotions may come up, sometimes very intensely. Kum Nye enables us to melt the qualities of all experiences, squeeze out the juice, and transform it into pure energy. Even qualities we may have been trained to restrain, such as passion, anger, and agitation, can be rich sources of energy. If we learn how to take away the words and dialogues, and stay with the energy itself, we can experience even this strong energy purely, as powerful vitality.

Kum Nye offers a way to support health, happiness, and inner peace, the foundation of meaning in life and the gateway to the most sublime meditative experience. Once we have internalized the experience of Kum Nye, we can carry it in our thoughts and allow it to brighten all that we see and hear. Kum Nye can lift our spirits with the joy of a beautiful day, with the sound of leaves rustling along a forest path, with the fragrance of flowers on a gentle breeze. Whatever kind of work we do, we can find ways to view it as a means of developing satisfaction. We can bring Kum Nye into all of our daily activities, taste the flavors of each experience, and blend their essence together into a rich nectar—a source of ongoing peace and happiness.

Although this may not be the ordinary Buddhist way, Kum Nye practices clearly reveal dimensions of experience concealed within the ordinary and routine. Even physical postures and movements can heal and energize at a very deep level, and this energy can manifest as qualities that begin to transform our way of being. The sharp edges that separate us from others begin to soften; we become more appreciative of our embodiment and respect the embodiment of others in a new light. Frustration melts into forbearance, and forbearance into patience.

In establishing this foundation, we gain some insight into our own spiritual qualities and how they can be further developed. As we mature in this practice, we may come to understand better the frustration and fears common to all human beings. Appreciating the benefits of Kum Nye, we may be inspired to share this knowledge with others. If so, the seeds of wisdom and compassion can take root and develop.

10

Re-engineering the System

Many people today do not seem to feel fully in charge of their lives. Expressions of frustration with obligations, pressure, and stressful conditions are heard ever more often in conversations and recorded in the media. Individuals from nearly all walks of life tend to voice their yearnings for vacations, solitude, or just more time to use as they please. Their time appears to be fully taken up, so tightly scheduled that there is little space for anything more in their lives.

In looking more closely at the background for all this activity, it becomes clear that the lives of most adults today have been tightly planned and scheduled since early childhood. The schedules can begin as early as two years of age. They intensify through grade and high school, as activities are added—different kinds of sports, lessons in dance or music, youth organizations, and other ways in which parents encourage children to develop their talents.

Scheduling continues as individuals take jobs or further educational goals through college, graduate school, and professional training. At the same time, activities become more complex and responsibilities more pressing. Deadlines are set and expectations have to be met. At some point they begin their life's work, and schedules and expectations become more demanding.

As adults, we feel the pressure of time nearly continually—and what time is available is already committed to a great many things that have to be done every day. We all have to sleep, eat, and take care of body functions; we all have to clean our living spaces, dress, socialize, and keep track of large amounts of information. For nearly everyone, still more time slips away here and there, in exercising emotions and dwelling on memories, anticipations, and worries that keep mind leaping from past to future and back again, competing with efforts to concentrate and accomplish. Then there are fears, expectations, feelings of inadequacy, and self-doubts—the negative thoughts that surface from time to time and tend to shadow us like a retinue.

The program is well established, and it keeps going on; every day, every week, month after month, year after year. If nothing happens to change it, most people will follow it to the end of their working lives. When their energy wanes and they can no longer keep up, they may well feel useless or unwanted, and lack the inner resources to support feelings of self-worth and satisfaction.

This is what Buddhism calls samsara, the busy yet aimless round of existence portrayed in paintings of the bhavacakra, or wheel of life. The wheel keeps turning, and people keep doing, bound up in endless variations on the same themes, one moment enjoying the fortunate realms of humans and gods, and the next suffering the miseries of the hells. But they, like ourselves, can never catch up with time; their time runs its course and new cycles begin. Our lives may not appear so dramatic, yet they seem to follow a similar pattern: The schedules are set, the program is running, and our time is occupied and driven by the needs of the pattern. We have no time for ourselves. We have no time to be.

Yet worry, guilt, fear, and pressures continue to steal time from more productive and happier pursuits. Many people today find it difficult to cope; caught in unhappy situations and seeing no way out, bounded by social conventions and restrictions on one side and guilt and regrets on the other, it is easy to feel hopeless and overwhelmed. When this happens, fear attacks the mind, anxiety strikes at the heart, and panic creates knots in the stomach. Filled with thoughts and feelings that cannot be expressed, the mind slips into despair.

Evaluating the System

Most of us would probably agree that nervous tension, agitation, and pain are signs that the body system is not stable and our energy is not circulating in a steady, balanced way. Emotions and perceptions that pop up from nowhere also indicate that something is disturbing us and causing our energy to percolate and bubble up erratically. The Buddha and the great Arhats, able to perfectly regulate their breath and balance their physical systems, did not have such disturbances. Their vital energies (vayu), self-renewing and free of dependence on anything external, sustained them in perfect bliss. Although vayu is most commonly translated as energy, vayu has a wide range of subtle meanings that the word energy cannot adequately express.

In the Ayurvedic system, vayu refers to the vital energy that enters the body as breath and flows throughout the body along channels known as nadi (nerves, blood vessels, and the central vital channels of the subtle body). Vayu enables speech, strengthens mind and memory, and sustains other vital functions, while nadi link the energy centers (cakras) of crown, forehead, throat, heart, and navel and all their associated organs and fields of operation. While there are five different kinds of vayu related to heart, lungs, circulatory, renal, digestive, excretory, and other systems, the principal vayu is associated with breath. Breath is the primary vehicle of mental and physical vitality.

The nadi system of nerves works much like a radar dish: its field extends outward in all directions, searching for stimulations, data it can read out, record, and instantaneously transmit. As impulses are cognized and identified, associations made, and memories and projections take form, a tremendous volume of input and output flash back and forth to and from cakras, brain, and senses with electrical speed. But all this data, in various stages of manipulation, travels back and forth along the same pathway. Confusion and overload is almost built into our systems, and our fast-paced way of life intensifies the stress.

Just as most people who use computers do not know their history or how their parts are engineered or their circuits wired and interconnected, we have only superficial understanding of the subtle workings of the cakras, vayu, and nadi systems of our bodies. Our physical, mental, and emotional systems have developed somewhat haphazardly, in the context of conditions over which we often had little control. Most of the knowledge that has determined our patterns of thought, our conceptual structures, and the orientations of our minds came to us from others, and only rarely did our nerves, feelings, and emotions receive much attention or guidance.

Although we did not plan our inner architecture, its structures are firmly in place: connections between senses and energy centers, energy centers and their fields of perception, perceptions and cognition, cognition and interpretation, feelings, and meaning and so on are now well established. Patterns have formed that tend to operate automatically, but, as we know from personal experience, the architecture itself may not hold up under all conditions. Imbalances and upsets are inevitable, but lacking knowledge of their root cause, we have difficulty understanding what has happened and regaining a sense of control.

Pain and suffering may be good teachers, but negativity can be a very unpleasant and exhausting curriculum. It can squeeze the enjoyment out of life, and even cripple us emotionally and intellectually. While we may not like to think of ourselves as bound to a program, we seem to be conditioned in ways that make us vulnerable to negativity. We may not be able to perceive alternatives, and our choices are limited. But if we knew the source code—if we understood how our energy centers function, how all their fields of perception were interconnected, and the way readouts happen—we would understand how to connect the parts and make the energy flow smoothly through our systems. Seeing where adjustments were needed, we could reverse engineer the program and redesign it to accord better with who we are and support our ability to accomplish what we wish with our lives. Then we, not the programming, would be in control, and we would be able to tune the engines of our body systems more effectively.

It is not too late to open a space in our tight, pressured lives so we can make a new home and create a new life. When we know how to relax completely, we can rest in the realm of joy and bliss, where we can evaluate all the elements of the program objectively.Then we can gain the knowledge we need to shape it in positive ways and establish more control of our time and our lives.

Change the Program!

Senses, nerves, cakras, breath, and mind work together to generate a continual flow of experience. The senses receive stimuli, the nerves transmit them, the cakras connect them with our vital organs; the breath vitalizes the body systems, and the mind identifies and interprets. Each of these has established its own pattern, and changing these patterns will require our attention and the dedication to remind ourselves frequently.

Each of our senses has properties that can be gentled, balanced, and attuned to relaxation. Kum Nye exercises work with the breath to develop each of the senses in turn. Attention to the simple act of inhaling and exhaling will begin to stimulate the flow of feeling that refreshes and opens the senses. As the senses open, they bring more pleasant feelings that carry us into deeper relaxation. Fresh, expansive energy courses through body and mind, dispelling pressure and transforming tension into bliss. It radiates outward as creative energy, opening pathways to new knowledge.

While the senses can initiate and support this process, the key to change and transformation lies in the mind. It is mind that organizes sensory information and shapes it into a wide range of expressions, from perceptions, thoughts, and views to desires, agitation, anger, love, and all other feelings and emotions. For mind to give us more pleasurable perceptions, interpretations, and thoughts, all aspects of our physical being—including vayu, nadi, cakras, and senses—have to be tuned individually and made to work together harmoniously. For this to happen, we need to work with the mind.

Mind moves quickly, even when relaxed, and a restless and tense mind can be as shy and reactive as a wild horse. At the outset, we may have to soothe and quiet it, so it is not distracted by emotionality, game-playing, or neurotic compulsions. When the mind becomes calm, it naturally becomes more accommodating, more sensitive to our needs and more creative in its support. Then it can process sensory information more fully, heal the pathways that lead to confusion and emotionality, and present us with clearer courses of action. Supported by mind's genius for coordinating and structuring the resources of nadi, vayu, cakras, and senses, it is possible for us to take charge of our lives more directly. Even in times of highly charged emotional distress, we can calm our minds, restore balance, and open our hearts to joyful feelings.

Kum Nye relaxes the senses and gives ease to the mind, relieving emotionality and providing the openness mind needs to establish new connections and create a new way of being. It cuts through the inner dialogues and dramas of artificial existence and connects us with the living pulse of real time, the source of confidence that comes from the center of our being. It replaces the pressure of shoulds and woulds, the restrictions and obligations imposed from outside, with an inner discipline grounded in knowledge, good feelings, and goodwill. Mind and perceptions feel clean and clear—our whole being is brighter and more joyous. We are happy, free at last of secret fears, no longer so vulnerable to feelings of unworthiness or rejection. We can breathe more freely, as if we had acquired a spacious new home with beautiful vistas, filled with light and the fragrance of incense and flowers.

11

Tuning Our Physical Senses

Our senses open doors to the world around us. Fully attuned to the present moment, they invite us to participate in a world alive with the rhythms of light, color, texture, shape, fragrance, taste, and sound, ever changing, ever new, an ongoing celebration of life. As their presentations pulse through our nerves and vital centers, feelings surge through our bodies like music, with tones that merge and blend to become our experience. The more complete the sensations, the richer the feelings; the deeper the flow of feeling, the more profound the experience. Subtle, yet tightly held tensions melt; the gates to meaning open wide, transforming our understanding of love and compassion and conveying the quiet joy of contentment.

The power of the senses to fill the being with bliss was known to the siddhas and great Arhats, who could sustain themselves in rarified states of rapture for very long periods of time. In the West, we have lost touch with this part of our human heritage and may not now appreciate or comprehend the fullness of experience. Perhaps we are too preoccupied with thoughts, worries, and plans, with shoulds and should nots, with have tos and wants.

We look at, but do we see? We hear, but how well? Of all the sensations that flow through our being each day, how many can we remember?

Our senses open outward, and we experience the results of their activity. We would not want to lose any one of them, yet we rarely give much thought to them or appreciate what joy and beauty they can give us. Perhaps because they are so intimately a part of our being, we tend to take them for granted. Ignorant of their needs, unaware of the abundance of joy they can bring to our lives, we abuse and deprive them. Closed and tight, starved for nourishment, they now tend to respond more fully to pain than to pleasure.

Relax and Heal

Kum Nye is a way to relax and heal the gates of the senses, so that they also open inward, transmitting the full richness of experience and bringing more pleasure and joy into our lives. Kum Nye enables us to relax deeply and to be fully within the flow of sensory experience. When we do this, the senses soften their focus on externals and reveal what is before us in greater clarity and depth. A sense of intimacy develops that eases our restlessness and satisfies our hunger for meaning. If we take every opportunity to nourish the senses with love and appreciation, they will reward us with a continual flow of blessings that deepen into a reliable source of contentment and meaning.

The six sense organs—eye, ear, nose, tongue, body, and mind—are important gateways for different kinds of experiences. Each of the six senses has its own faculty; each faculty has its distinctive character and field of operation. As we respond to experience, each faculty operates within its own territory, recording relevant data and shaping it into meaning. To get the maximum benefit from each moment of experience, we need to develop the full potential of each of our senses. So it is important to focus on exercising at least one of the six senses for forty-five minutes daily. If you spend two weeks on each of the senses in turn, you may notice a clear improvement in the quality of your perceptions.

Engage All Seasons and Situations

Which seasons and environments do you find most attractive and accommodating? Do you yearn to spend time in the forest or jungle, on beaches, near lakes and oceans, or do you feel more at home in the mountains or desert? Whether you have strong preferences or can adapt to any kind of environment, you will benefit greatly from loosening up fixed attitudes and engaging all seasons and situations freshly (unless you have limitations that make this inadvisable). For example, even if you are not fond of city life, you can benefit from short periods of immersion in the stimulating dynamic of an urban environment. If you are not comfortable with open spaces, silence, and lack of modern conveniences, it can be helpful to suspend your judgments and preferences and spend some time in the rural countryside.

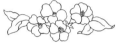

12

The Six Senses: Visual - Eye

Normally, when we look around us, we see objects that we recognize and can name. This kind of response has become so automatic that we rarely have reason to consider just how we see and examine more closely the process of seeing. Although most of this process unfolds below the horizon of our conscious awareness, when we slow it down, we can break it into stages that may give us some insight into how eye and mind work together to establish our sense of reality. First comes light, then awareness of shapes and forms that we recognize through associations with past experiences. Although we may not be familiar with a specific form that is presenting itself to the eye, we immediately associate it with a range of labels and classifications that we have already learned to accept, and we settle on the one that seems most appropriate at that particular time. For instance, a form has a shape I have learned to associate with flowers and it appears in an environment where a flower might be expected. Instantly I identify it as a flower. I may not be familiar with its color, size, shape of petals, chemical properties, or other details, but I understand that it is a flower. In the same way, we recognize a table, chair, or tool the instant the eye connects with an object that we have learned to identify as very similar.

We have named the object, so now we have a general idea of what it is. Often that general idea is sufficient. Once the primary impulse to identify the object has served its purpose, the energy of perception tends to wane, and the eye moves on to another object. But very little information has actually been transmitted; the perceptive impulse has not been strong enough to imprint on our memory or to stimulate a response. Of the innumerable objects perceived in any one day, how many can we actually remember?

The very speed of our visual perception enables us to take in a wealth of information at a glance. Yet the eye jumps so quickly from one object to another that we rarely benefit fully from what its impressions convey. We may not know exactly what we are looking at, but we make assumptions based on what we have been told or experienced. This pattern has been developed and transmitted for centuries and now operates nearly automatically. As a result, most people take countless objects for granted: this is a horse, a car, a train; that is a man, a woman, a child; those are stars, that is the moon, that is the sun; these are books, this is food. There is no need to analyze or question further: nothing more needs to be said.

If something about an object catches and holds our attention, more information may come through and awaken our interest, for instance, in what a person does or knows or in how an object operates. Something about a flower may inspire our going further to find out what kind of flower it is, what climate is most favorable for it, and what are its characteristics. We begin to perceive differences and wonder about their purpose or usefulness; we notice how a person moves and speaks; we note intensities of color and the play of light and shadow.

Sustained contact with the object tends to call forth additional information as we notice more details and identify it more precisely. Contact and associations with past experiences give rise to feelings of various intensity: we want or we don't want the object; we like it or we do not like it, or we feel neutral, having no strong opinions either way. For example, what we thought might be an interesting vine turns out to be poison oak, and we respond with distaste or revulsion. Or, when we identify a person as a friend, qualities and experiences we associate with friendship spring to mind, and our attitudes and behavior follow from that set of associations.

Users, Not Knowers

Most of us are not accustomed to thinking about objects in a sophisticated, analytic way. We tend to take what we see at face value: we recognize, then accept the name of the object, but often there is no impulse to look more closely and perceive additional details. The observer may recognize a table, but not notice the kind of wood the table is made of, where the wood comes from, the quality of the workmanship, the details of its design, or consider other possible uses for this specific form. A computer or television may have many interesting parts and a long history of technical development; it can organize flows of electrons to project images in billions of colors and access information from all over the globe, but we normally do not grasp the significance of these more sophisticated aspects. It has a function, and we can use it. But we do not really know it.

Similarly, once an object has been introduced, most individuals think there is nothing more to do. It is as if a person introduced himself, saying "My name is John." Then you can say, "This is John." John and the form you are seeing cannot be separated. From then on, the form is identified. "This is John." This kind of identification is very much the same as saying "This is a table." Once the object is pointed out, it is a table. We know it is a table, because we have accepted that the name "table" applies to this object. But we do not really know this table.

The eye contacts an object and projects the image to consciousness. Consciousness clicks on the object as if taking a picture, and then moves on. We identify the surface form instantly, "This is my friend." "Those are my parents," but we may not notice any further details. For example, the eye sees a beautiful rainbow, so we accept that the rainbow exists, that it is something real and solid. The eye does not notice that the background is empty space, or that the colors of the rainbow are refractions of light waves passing through mist. It simply sees and accepts what presents itself, as if the rainbow were somehow painted in space.

Characteristics and distinctions come immediately—beautiful, ugly, tall, or short; I like it, I don't like it—along with associations, opinions, and judgments: fun, love, guilt, noisy, quiet, comfort, security, warm, cold. We use language to give everything an identity and endow it with characteristics and associations. We do not know why we use these words for this shape and form; they just come to mind and we accept them automatically—this is what the object is. We have no other way to think about it. Very little in this process leads to adjusting or deepening our initial perception: "things are what they are." Familiar objects are essentially frozen in consciousness, along with associations and assumptions.

Squeezed and pressured in these ways, our eye consciousness has become too jumpy and erratic to allow awareness to operate steadily. Dialogues and other distractions that pop into mind increase this jumpiness. Many people today seek nearly continual sensory stimulation, and there is little in modern life that encourages us to be quiet, to seek solitude and relax. So we may not notice that our visual senses might be capable of far more than we realize. The eye has a special affinity for light; awareness related to the eye illumines space and allows us to see shape and form; it connects with the tissues of the brain, opening a window that gives us access to a universe of unimaginable beauty. Before our eyes manifests an ever-shifting kaleidoscope of shapes and forms, an ongoing exhibition that gives interest and meaning to life. Exercises that nourish the faculties related to eye and eye-consciousness can awaken the light of awareness; simple, yet magical and uplifting, they can transform the quality of our lives.

Opening and Relaxing:
1 Just Seeing

Sitting quietly, choose something you find pleasant to look at. Perhaps the color of something around you attracts your eye, or you notice a natural form, such as a flower or a tree. Gaze softly at the color and form, letting your attention trace the contours of the shape and vibrate with the energy of the color. Gradually, you will sense the color and form very simply.

If you wish, you could look at a traditional symbol sometimes used in meditation, such as the Tibetan letter A. With your attention, trace the outline of the form, starting at the top left corner and ending with the top right corner.

As you sit longer with just seeing, note areas of tension within the body and relax them one by one, until your body feels loose and comfortable. The eyes too will relax their tendencies to stare at the object and look more gently, observing, but not necessarily focusing on it. Even the attention tracing the shape gradually relaxes into the feeling of the shape.

Simply be aware that the object or meditation letter is there; see it in its entirety, without paying attention to specific details or seeking to grasp or understand it. Any effort to think about, analyze, or interpret the object directs your senses outward in a grasping way and constricts awareness. There is nothing specific that you need to do. Just remain quiet and relaxed, and allow what is before you to present itself. Any tension that remains will eventually relax, and you will experience the openness of simply seeing. If you have difficulty understanding this meditative way of seeing, you can ease into it by just softening the eyes and looking more gently, not necessarily focusing on anything. Develop this practice in sessions of twenty to twenty-five minutes twice each day for at least one week.

As much as possible, as you go about your daily activities, be aware when your eyes are open that they are not "hunter's eyes," looking with strong, outward-directed focus for whatever they can catch. From time to time, close your eyes a few moments, relax them, then open them, and invite the light to come into your awareness in a calm, meditative manner. Then carry the feeling of relaxed ease into your next activity.

At first objects that present themselves to you are solid and real. They have form, shape, and color—physical qualities and characteristics you can definitely see. You may give little thought to space at this point, for, on this fundamental level, you know you cannot see space; space is empty, without any distinct characteristics that the senses can directly perceive. The eye goes straight to forms, and the mind follows. You can infer the existence of space, for without space you would not be able to distinguish forms. But you do not tend to interpret what you see as space that happens to be surrounding some solid objects. When reflecting further on how you relate to form and space, and allowing your practice to unfold over time, a fresh way of seeing may present itself. You may understand that there is ultimately no difference between space and the object that manifests within it. The distinction between form and the surrounding space no longer separates the two. Form may be perceived as space, and space as form. Understanding how this works is the key to developing your visual capacities further.

2 Opening Seeing

Continue to relax, with eyes focusing lightly, and allow opportunity for stillness to develop. You may experience a softening sensation in the eyes, a gentling and calming quality. Whatever feelings come up, allow them to expand and relax deeply into them, until you are no longer the one seeing—there is only seeing.

As the eyes relax, more light enters, illumining awareness and inviting a quality of openness and pleasure in the simple act of seeing. With your eyes more fully open and seeing in a less forced, more neutral manner, your concentration and awareness become more steady. You may have a sense of light in, around, or behind the image, even if you cannot actually see light itself.

As relaxation continues to deepen, seeing takes on a gentler and more allowing quality that is not so tightly bound to I, me, or mine. As the sense of subject/object lessens, the edges of the image you are viewing may become less distinct, possibly translucent or even transparent. Continue to develop this exercise by practicing it for twenty to twenty-five minutes twice a day for two weeks.

3 Panoramic Seeing

When you begin to understand the interconnection of light and awareness, you can more easily soften tendencies to look at objects and allow them to simply be in your field of awareness. One day you may realize that you are not even focusing on a particular object. You may note your perception taking on a more rounded, three-dimensional aspect and become more aware of the relationship of objects and space. At some point, you may sense the field of awareness expanding to encompass all objects panoramically, as if you were looking at the reflection of a thousand stars in a pool of water, seeing each one distinctly, yet all of them simultaneously. It is important to exercise this capacity and develop it to the fullest.

As your practice continues, you may find that seeing merges with meditation: seeing becomes meditation, and meditation becomes seeing. This meditative seeing connects with objects in a different way. Day or night, objects are seen as having a luminous light quality; they lose their solidity and appear almost translucent. Experiencing objects in this way transforms your way of being, softening judgmental and critical tendencies and allowing more openness for compassion and skillful action.

Eventually you may come to understand how awareness related to the eye enables you to perceive qualities inherent in objects around you, but that now pass you by without your noticing. Among them are dimensions of beauty: perfections of shape, color, movement, and proportions that can enrapture the mind, unfolding layers of meaning and purpose. Uplifted by beauty and attuned to deeper purposes, consciousness transforms. From this foundation, it is possible to benefit from the oral instructions of a qualified teacher, who can transmit the profound meanings encoded in mandalas and symbols. In time, if you continue to develop this capacity, you may come to embody these meanings directly. Then you may understand what is meant by the phrase, Liberation Through Seeing.

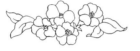

13

Sound - Ear

Sounds come to us continually through the media of voice and music as well as through the operation of natural forces and man-made machinery. Some sounds are pleasant and reassuring; some are distracting, unpleasant, frightening, or even painful. Sounds convey meaning: we hear the messages they convey and react to them with actions, judgments, and opinions. But we rarely focus on the inner quality of sound itself. In overlooking the silent center of sound, we lose touch with the full range of meaning that sounds convey.

Kum Nye exercises can enhance sensitivity to sound, revealing the power of sound to evoke ecstatic experiences and open new dimensions of significance concealed within ordinary experience. We can develop this sensitivity by setting aside likes and dislikes and taking opportunities to work with all kinds of sound. Anytime a sound comes into our consciousness, we can use it as an exercise and go into it in this contemplative way.

When we relax our hold on the meanings of sound and no longer judge and discriminate, sound takes on the quality of silence. Hearing continues, but sound itself is silent. Listening in this way, we can gradually transform our understanding of sound and the relationship of sound to meaning. This practice develops our ability to hear subtleties of meaning beyond what words can express. This ability is useful in conversation and other kinds of intellectual activity.

Stages of Opening:
1 Simply Hearing

Chant AH or the Vajra Guru Mantra. First, listen to your own voice and contemplate the sound. Follow the sound as it goes far away, into the distance, further out to infinity, yet still not stopping. The words trail away and whatever meanings you may have assigned to them fade, but the sound remains, resonating in your awareness and vibrating deep in your inner ear. Practice following the sound as long as you can in this way for twenty-five repetitions.

A bell or a singing bowl can be used in the same way. The sound itself may be complex, with beats and overtones, but it has no words for the mind to grasp onto. Listen to the sound, feel its quality vibrating deep in your inner ear and in the nerves leading to your brain. Relax as completely as possible as the sound starts to fade; follow the sound as it slips away, then follow the feeling of the sound as it continues to resonate in your consciousness. Follow it deep into silence, then sit quietly for ten to fifteen minutes.

2 Panoramic Hearing

Follow the sound going out into one direction, toward a far distant point. Then imagine the sound going out into three directions, and follow all three streams of sound as far as you can. Finally, follow the sound as it goes out and away, moving outward to all directions simultaneously, like rings rippling out from a waterfall to shores far beyond. Develop these sound exercises as much as you can.

3 Silence of Sound

After you can follow the sound into all directions, you may note subtle changes in the silence that follows it. As the sensing tension of the ears relaxes, you may notice the silence as a clear open space, perhaps somewhat luminous and inviting. If pleasant feelings arise, follow them into that space and feel the space expanding with each exhalation. The quality of sound may continue going on, even within the silence, almost like a memory. Just let it be. Let silence, sound, and feeling melt together.

Sound and Meaning

In the West, particularly, individuals reflexively join sound and meaning to analyze what is said. Sound carries the words, and words carry meaning and give feedback that can be evaluated and judged. If we fail to notice a transition between sound, words, and meaning, it may seem as though meaning relies on words that can be pronounced or written down. Without words, it may seem as though sound has no meaning. Yet, from another perspective, sound is the carrier of meaning. Meaning is introduced through our sense of hearing and our ability to understand the forms that express it, whether these forms consist of words, music, or sounds produced through other means.

When we consider the relationship between words, sound, and meaning, we can see that meaning conveyed through words ultimately depends on sound. Sound is essential for meaning to be vocalized, and meaning can be communicated directly through sound itself. For example, blessings can be conveyed through the chanting of ceremonies, and different levels of meaning can be expressed simultaneously in the chanting of dharanis. Yet those who rely primarily on words may have difficulty understanding how communication of meaning can transcend the specific associations of words.

Words and meanings stimulate each other, interacting to build up our understanding of reality. Any words we speak are conveying meaning—all our conversations, real or imagined; all our inner dialogues and speech heard or expressed in dreams. These meanings feed back to our consciousness, where they are recorded. Even if we do not hear the sound that is carrying these words, the sound is always there. These sounds are connected with our hearing faculty; they are imprinted in our consciousness, which is why we can hear the words and associate them with meaning.

Practicing Kum Nye sound exercises can extend our awareness of sound as having significance in itself. We may also begin to appreciate the relationship of sound and words, even when sound manifests subtly, as it does in conversation. Awareness developed through hearing opens up new dimensions of meaning that enable us to distinguish more clearly between what is real and not real, what is true and what is not true. This knowledge can strengthen confidence and enrich our lives with continual streams of joy and appreciation.

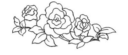

14

Feeling - Body

Our fundamental human expressions—joy, love, eating, resting, comfort-seeking, sadness, numbness, excitement, exhilaration, even deep depression—are closely related to the body and its capacity for feeling. Of all our sensory properties, feelings may be our most important. Their tones resonate continually through our bodies, stimulated by our mental and sensory perceptions, and each kind of feeling has its specific character and power. Some are neutral, or so gentle that we may not notice them; others—as when we feel good or bad—affect our attitudes and actions more strongly. Still others—the more volatile emotions—can be so intense as to be uncontrollable. Their energies can flash through the body with electrical speed, constricting the navel, heart, and throat cakras, throwing thoughts into disarray, and distorting sensory perceptions. When strong feelings range out of control, the urge to respond can be overwhelming. Exhilaration, love, and joyous rapture can prompt impulsive and even extreme responses; grief can override the will to live; anger and hatred can blind us to our own best interests; and depression can blacken consciousness and paralyze our ability to act.

Feelings can be rich and nourishing, vital pathways to a deep and abiding joy that calms the mind, balances the ups and downs of life, and stabilizes us in the midst of difficulties. Yet we do not seem able to manage our feelings well. Too often we are influenced by pressures and negativity assaulting us from within and without, feeding fears and insecurities and heightening feelings of isolation and hopelessness. We do our best to suppress the harsher effects of negative thoughts and emotions, but ultimately it seems we have little control over what we feel or do not feel. Our bodies bear residues of negative emotions; pressures accumulate in our organs, robbing them of vitality, and tension takes hold deep in muscles and circulatory systems. Perhaps out of despair or desperation, many individuals intensify their difficulties by taking refuge in extremes. Even those who appear to be doing well may be inwardly impoverished, unable to feel deeply, and out of touch with the joy and creativity that gives life meaning.

It is vitally important that we cultivate a stronger sense of feeling and learn to direct these powerful energies in positive ways. Kum Nye exercises can help us change our inner architecture from the ground up, loosening the body, refreshing the senses, and brightening the mind. Wherever we are, whatever we are doing, we can connect mindfully with the feelings that are resonating in the body at that particular moment. Whatever feeling we notice, we can listen for its tone, gently touching it with our breath, and allowing it to expand as far as possible. Breathing lightly, we can melt into the center of the feeling and rest in that inner silence.

1 Relieving Pressure

From time to time, when you feel pressured and frustrated, strong emotions may cause you to act in ways you might later regret. Now, with intense energy coursing through your body, is when you need to practice Kum Nye and embody it as fully as possible. Breathing softly through nose and mouth, relax your throat, chest, and abdomen, and allow your breathing to slow to a natural rhythm. Observe the breath moving smoothly in and out of the body, touching the agitation and helping it settle down. As you follow the movement of the breath, you may notice breath and feeling coming together, then merging into a single sensation. Gradually, breath and feeling become open and light, like space. Body and mind lighten and become calm, completely relaxed. You are not holding on to anything, not to feelings or sensations, not to external objects, and nothing is holding on to you.

2 Calming Intense Energy

Kum Nye can smooth out the wild, almost uncontrollable surge of exhilaration and transform it into a deep and steady flow of feeling. It can also stabilize strong reactive tendencies and transform the energy they stimulate from negativity into ecstatic bliss. This practice can become a reliable source of healing for both body and mind, a foundation for meditation and a source of inner freedom.

Breathing through nose and mouth, relax into the feelings as much as possible. If the strong energy of exhilaration stimulates a current of thoughts, breathe into the current and let the thoughts stream by. As feelings arise, touch them gently with the breath, gather them together, and let them ride on the flow of breath. Without thinking about who is getting the experience, taste the feelings and savor them deeply. Let them nourish the heart with aliveness.

Using the flow of breath, turn up your inner heat and intensify the feelings—really get into them and be with that strong energy as it peaks. Then completely relax. Let everything go and surrender completely to the experience. Without focusing on anything, just BE. Let your entire being become openness—just breath moving back and forth through empty space. Stay with that relaxation for twenty to thirty minutes, allowing the breath to become slow and light.

Merged with awareness of space, the energy of exhilaration flows through heart, body, and senses like amrita, the nectar of immortality, relaxing the force of thoughts and melting the bonds of ego. Likes and dislikes, accepting and rejecting, judgments of good and bad all melt and become one with the bliss flooding your being.

When you are able to stay in this energized state of relaxation for twenty to thirty minutes at a time, feelings of relief and joy may begin arising spontaneously, not only during your practice, but also in your work and other daily activities. Eventually, you may become aware of a new, more vital sense of love that seems to come from deep within your being. You feel good about yourself and see others in a gentler, more compassionate light. You are not so quick to judge their actions or feel defensive when they challenge you. As love grows in your heart, it expands in all directions, embracing others and nourishing yourself.

As you practice, you can touch your memory of blissful feelings and bring them alive in the present. This will calm and satisfy the mind, and the mind will cooperate by relaxing gently into meditation.

3 Allowing Feeling to Touch Meditation

Eventually, you will find that whatever feelings are present, whether soft or strong, you can relax into them and allow them to merge and come into balance. Breathing through both nose and mouth, sense your breath floating gently on top of the current of feeling, rising and sinking slightly as you inhale and exhale. If the underlying feeling-tones are agitated or sad, touch memories of beauty, and allow those feelings to merge gently into your feeling-stream. When the feelings lighten, touch memories of joy, and bring those feelings into your stream also. Let the stream of feeling broaden and expand, gradually broadening out into space. Follow it with the breath, breathing into space, until even the sense of feeling dissipates and there is only space.

Eventually you will be able to lighten and direct feelings at will. At this point, if you wish to go further into meditation, you should seek the guidance of an experienced teacher who is well-grounded in a meditative lineage.

15

Taste - Tongue

Taste has a tactile reality associated with touch and nurturing. Mouth touching breast, opening to receive milk flowing through the nipple, is one of human's earliest experiences. It establishes a strong bond with the parent or caregiver, a sense of connection that we continue to express by offering food as gestures of hospitality and friendship. When we practice Kum Nye, we can draw upon this association to feed the senses and spirit and nourish a stronger interconnection among all aspects of our being.

Many individuals, too pressured and tense to enjoy the preparation and relishing of food, may tend to regard eating as a kind of duty. Hunger has an anxious quality that begs for satisfaction, and it is not possible to ignore it. Yet we seem to be losing touch with how to satisfy hunger in a way that gives pleasure and nourishes our whole being. Many respond nearly reflexively, looking for something that will ease these sensations with very little attention to what they are doing. For some, the connection between hunger and eating may become so automatic that they may not even remember having eaten. Others may deny their hunger and attempt to redirect the cravings that accumulate. When hunger is denied or goes unsatisfied, its nagging quality continues and tends to spread to other areas of our lives.

1 An Offering of Taste

All the food we eat, all the liquids we drink go through the mouth and are felt and savored by taste buds located along the edge of the tongue. These tactile sensations can encourage us to nourish ourselves in a deeper, more satisfying way.

Consider food as an offering to your own body, mind, and senses. Prepare food as if you were preparing offerings for a ceremony, being mindful of each step in the process. Work as silently as possible, staying focused on the textures and colors of the foods you are handling, with no extraneous conversation.

When the food is ready and placed on the table, the ceremony begins. Sit in a balanced, relaxed way. Allow the breath to become balanced and even. If you wish, chant OM AH HUM slowly three times, making one complete exhalation as you chant each syllable. Sit quietly a few moments, and then begin the meal. Offer food to yourself in a joyful and respectful manner. Feel the texture and taste of the food in the mouth and on the tongue; savor the taste—

does it come all at once? Is there a single taste, or does one follow another? Does the taste intensify as you breathe in? Does it change as you exhale? Practice touching each taste gently throughout the meal and savor the feelings of pleasure that arise and spread throughout your body. Do this at least once a day for several weeks.

2 Healing Taste of Kum Nye

When you become more sensitive to the tactile qualities of food preparation and enjoyment, you can intensify the pleasure of tasting by easing into flavors more fully and sensitively. As you notice a taste, stay with it—Is it sweet, sour, salty, or bitter, or a combination? Taste it carefully—there may be many layers of flavor there, and the tongue may be capable of picking up more of them than you have been able to notice before.

Each layer of flavor connects with nerves that can send messages of relaxation and pleasure throughout the body. Reach out to these flavors, breathe in their essence, drink their juice. Taste them in the lining of your mouth, on the edges and back of your tongue. Sense their essence entering your body, sending ripples of pleasurable feelings through the nerves of the tongue. Allow these feelings to penetrate deeply into the body, connecting the cakras and bathing them in the gentle warmth of healing energy.

3 Nourishing Your Being

As your senses become more attuned to the pleasurable sensations of taste, your ability to sink into them deeply will increase. At this point, feelings can relax you more deeply and lead you to meditation. Continue to take food and drink in a mindful, relaxed way, swallowing and drinking, breathing naturally, and relishing taste and texture. Notice the kind of tastes you are savoring. Make each taste more distinct; gently touch one after the other, creating a mandala of flavor—an offering for transforming your body. Breathe in the flavor, sense it in both nostrils and mouth, and savor it as deeply as possible. If pleasurable feelings come, breathe into them; intensify them as much as possible, and follow them as they fade away. In the calm that follows, nourishment permeates the entire body like a transforming elixir; the whole body becomes part of these substances.

Exercise this kind of Kum Nye as much as you can during meals.

When you apply this Kum Nye practice mindfully, day after day, the now mundane task of food preparation and eating can become a ceremony, an offering of appreciation for this precious human embodiment. This practice can help restore a sense of wholeness that we may have been missing a long time.

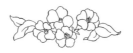

16

Smell - Nose

Scents and fragrances enter the body on the current of the breath: we notice and identify them almost immediately as pleasant or foul. Passing through the nostrils, they activate the olfactory glands that connect directly to the brain and stimulate a specific area of the brain that other senses cannot reach. Almost immediately, this activity creates an entire environment, awakening the nerves of eye, ear, tongue and stimulating thoughts and associations in the mind.

Good smells inspire and delight; they can release tension and call forth fond memories, brighten attitudes, and transform an indifferent or negative mind into a pleasant and inviting field of experience. The eye might perceive images of open fields or specific kinds of flowers; the ear might be reminded of the sound of wind in the trees, and the tongue might anticipate some delicious taste. Even if no associations have yet developed for a specific fragrance, or the fragrance is new and unfamiliar, its scent can relax the nerves and loosen up the body.

Dirty, stale-smelling, or messy surroundings oppress the senses, lower our sense of confidence and self-esteem, and depress our motivation, while fresh, clean smells brighten and calm the mind, lightening feelings and thoughts. Nature has a powerful healing quality, not only through the beauty of its creations but also through the energy of the smells that pervade the natural environment, especially the scents of flowers and trees. These fragrances are nature's gift to us, conveyed through the air and presented freely to us as a precious treasure. Flowers communicate an immediacy of life and vitality that uplifts and refreshes. They awaken appreciation and make us feel good. So it is important for our sense of well-being to refresh our living and working areas from time to time with fresh flowers, incense, and other pleasant fragrances.

1 Attuning to Fragrance

Dedicate an hour in the course of your daily activities when you can pay close attention to the smells of your surroundings. Start with familiar surroundings of home or office, or perhaps outside. Simply note the quality of fragrance and the feeling tones that different fragrances stimulate. Breathe deeply for a few breaths, then allow your breathing to settle into a slow, relaxed movement. When feelings come up, stay with them, letting go of associations and images. You can do this while seated or while standing or walking.

2 Fragrance and Feeling

Practice attention to fragrance whenever you find yourself in different surroundings—in gardens, beside a river, lake, or ocean, in the mountains, in cities, in different seasons and at different times of the day. Allow your awareness to touch the fragrance lightly. Note the connection between fragrance and memories, between fragrance and feelings. Just note how they connect, without dwelling on specific memories or feelings. Then relax deeply into the feelings. These exercises can be done while you are standing or walking.

Certain parts of the world have trees and plants that communicate distinctive qualities and create unusually attractive and beneficial environments, as if they had been prepared by the nagas to demonstrate the wondrous powers of nature. This is why meditating in a forest can instill such a strong sense of peace and tranquility. It is good to locate such special places where you are able to feel especially open and at ease, where you can enjoy the pleasures of the senses and experience deep enjoyment. Walk where fresh air can touch your body, washing away tension and stress, where earthy fragrances can give pleasure and bring up good memories, and where awareness of the abundance of life can nourish your soul.

17

Mind and Perceptions

When we contemplate without focusing on any specific object, we can observe the shimmery quality of the mind at rest. Then eyes and ears begin to grasp for sight and sounds, sending a flow of raw sensory data through our nerves. Within moments, impulses begin to pop up, forming ripples on the calm surface of mind. The flow of data becomes more insistent: Ripples become surges and waves that flow into consciousness and take on shape and form. Almost instantly, shape and form are no longer naked, but fully clothed in meaning and embellished with layers of associations and judgments, likes and dislikes, want and don't want. Suddenly we are aware: the perceptions are clear and distinct, and we know what they mean from their characteristics. We can identify not only a woman, but can also gain a wealth of information from her clothing, manner, and hairstyle. We see a robe and recognize from its style and color a lama, priest, or nun. Similarly, every perception comes dressed in its own distinctive clothing, and we know from that clothing what the image means, what to expect from it, and how to respond. The view is established, the meanings determined, and the mind is made up. Once all the perceptual threads are tied up into a single knot, it is almost impossible to untie them, sort them out, and come to a different conclusion.

Perceptions Dictate Responses

From time to time, especially if something has gone wrong in our lives, we might wonder, "How did that happen?" But we have little knowledge of how the process of cause and effect works. The Abhidharma tradition offers a way of understanding the operations of mind by describing fifty-one, or sometimes seventy-five or more mental events. Activated by the stream of perceptions that flow through mind's treasury of memories and associations, these mental events follow each other like boxcars on a train. Each has its own cause, effect, and outcome, yet all are linked together, influencing and reinforcing each other.

Some perceptions are familiar, and some are not, but in general they are related enough to enable us to respond: we want, or don't want; we grasp or reject; or we are neutral, not particularly motivated to reach out or to turn away. Neutral responses can be either positive or negative. A positive neutral response is free of grasping—allowing us to experience the calm and openness of simply being. But neutral can also have a dull, dark, and heavy quality that binds the knots of perceptions, associations, and meanings more tightly and imprints them more deeply on our consciousness.

Each of these—perceptions, mental events, and attitudes—has its own character that urges for expression. Since consciousness carries on these characteristics, our perception and the feelings that result are closely attuned to them. When a characteristic manifests, mind and body have to obey, and they obey in ways associated with each one. When these characteristics are positive, mind and body may manifest love and joy. When the characteristics are negative, mind and body may manifest anger and rage or dullness and apathy. They may also find expression as depression or in feelings of being alienated, lost, and alone. Whatever feelings and emotions come up, we have to deal with them. They control our being, and we have no choice.

How We Identify with Feelings and Emotions

Feelings and emotions present themselves to us like a progression of television shows. But we have little control over the programming—it turns on in the morning and continues to run through the night. Depending on the ebb and flow of events, our shifting perceptions, and internal dialogues, we feel the rapturous pleasure of love, the dull stagnation of boredom, the ebullience of joy, the agitation of anxiety or frustration, the warm reassurance of happiness, the pain of disappointment or loss. We see, we observe, and the force of our perceptions casts us into the drama. The script has been already written: the emotional reactions are predictable, and we experience what our impulses dictate. Once we take ownership of the experience, once we say "I am happy," "I am angry," "I am sad," I and the experience become one: I cannot separate myself from my perceptions or my emotions, or make distinctions between myself and my responses.

"I am angry." "Who is angry?" "Me. I am angry." How many times a day does this pattern repeat? How often do we say "I am not happy," or "I am happy," or some variation on this pattern? Once we identify ourselves with the feeling or emotion, it fuses to our perception of "me" and all that "me" means to us. Although we say "my joy," "my sorrow," as if we were in control, as soon as we relate experience so closely to ourselves, we are bonded to it. The association persists in our mind, coloring our perception of our experience and of ourselves.

I Know What I Mean

"I am not happy." Although we may know conceptually that this statement refers to a feeling-tone that happens to be present at the moment, we have established the association of "I" and "not happy" because that is the way we have learned to use the language. If someone asks, "What do you mean when you say I?" those not trained in an analytic way of thinking are likely to say, "You know what I mean." This means that you both agree and no further explanation is necessary. There is unhappiness, and this unhappiness is somehow "I". This association bonds to the resulting perception: "I am unhappy."

If we continue to ask what the connection between "I" and unhappy means, the person questioned may be at a loss for words. "What else could it mean? You are unhappy." The meaning of "unhappy" has been effectively transferred from a passing feeling-tone to "I", where it will cast a shadow on one's sense of self for a long time.

Although we may not spell it out in a physical way or explain the meaning logically, we have followed a conceptual pattern of labeling a quality, and that label has activated long-accepted rules concerning how we believe. "I" exist, "I" am the director, the principal actor; "I" have a territory, in which things happen to "me" and where objects are "mine." Without establishing this territory, we would find it difficult to speak.

Although this territory operates in the physical realm, it is so strongly established that we extend it automatically as well into the abstract realm, where ideas or other objects we cannot see, hear, taste, smell, or touch are also related somehow to "I", "me", or "mine." Even these objects can call forth a strong sense of identity that reinforces our sense of "I am."

Mind's Hall of Mirrors

Senses project perceptions to mind; mind identifies the perceptions, associates them with meanings, and reflects them back to mind for further interpretations. This activity prompts a chain of inner dialogues; these dialogues build on themselves, repeating over and over until fresh perceptions spark the creation of new story lines. We seem to be observing this activity, as if we were the audience watching a drama being staged. Depending on how we relate to the drama, we like it, we don't like it, we feel neutral, or we experience a range of other emotions and responses. All this mental activity takes place in mind's own inner realm.

This kind of mental reflecting—objects to cognitions to identifications to associations to inner dialogues that in turn become more objects—goes on continually. The mind serves as a hall of mirrors for perceptions that develop into daytime fantasies, imaginations, anticipations, hopes, and fears; at night the process continues, feeding images and emotions back to us in reverie, dreams, and nightmares.

On one hand, it seems as if these reflections are leading us on an interesting journey, ruminating on the past, recording the present, projecting the future, and weaving it all together in colorful ways. Although this kind of trip is all in the mind, we tend to experience it as though it were real.

The Self-Contained Realm of "I"

We have to participate in this mental journey, because that is how we communicate. The realm of "I" is our own private world: Each time we say "I" or communicate with ourselves through inner dialogues, our perceptions and thoughts seem to be constantly traveling along the same track, hooked together as if they were passenger cars on a train. Each car has its own set of compartments that house different perceptions and experiences, but all of them are going along the same track. Inner dialogues and thoughts entertain themselves in this way, occupying the mind and making us feel busy, but most of this busyness is unfolding in the realm of imagination. Lonely people sometimes escape to that realm for a long time.

Power of Imagination

Imagination, perhaps our most powerful mental faculty, can play a prominent role in our self-contained mental realm. Intimately identified with the self, it is our private territory, our own reading of what is happening, our personal encyclopedia of knowledge. So closely is it bonded to the reality we know, to our history in depth, to the truth of what we are seeing, that it can become as real as if we were seeing it in physical form. A traditional tale illustrates this aspect of imagination:

A woman, living in a village near Benares, was so consumed by anger that she began to visualize herself as a tiger. Her concentration became so strong and steady that other people also began to see this tiger. Gradually, the tiger was seen entering and leaving the woman's house by more and more people. When several villagers living nearby disappeared, the rest of the villagers began avoiding the area, and finally left the region altogether. Eventually, people in the neighboring villages also became able to see the tiger, and they too abandoned their homes and moved far away, fearing that the tiger would attack them.

Many people play in the realm of imagination so often that they experience very little distinction between physical reality—what is actually going on at the moment— and the reality that is truly all in their minds. This inner activity can be a kind of mind-food; they may think they are in good company and getting something delicious, but they may only be eating alone. Since the food has no substance, it nourishes only the imagination. The illusion of well-being will eventually dissipate, leaving them vulnerable to depression.

While these mental projections are not necessarily grounded in objective reality, they seem so important that we have difficulty ignoring them. Arising in the mind, they activate a complex of sensations, feelings, and thoughts that burst into consciousness with a compelling sense of urgency. They can take on a reality of their own, weaving fantasies that can lead to obsession and paranoia.

Ultimately, however strongly we identify ourselves with "our" mind, it seems that mind tends to play games that can confuse and delude us, and we are not fully in charge of this mind. At some point, we need to question our relationship to mind: Is mind really mine? Or is mind my partner, my boss, or my foundation? If mind is the foundation of our knowledge, and if knowledge determines the quality of our lives, it is in our best interest to investigate the nature of this mind.

To understand mind, it is helpful to look beneath the patterns woven into mind and experience more directly the sensing aspect of mind. This exploration can serve as a kind of Kum Nye for the mind, a way to soften the present patterns of mind and glimpse other possibilities for perceiving, thinking, and being. Reflecting on a few problematic aspects of perception and communication can be a good place to begin.

Perceptions Fragmented

Ideally, sensory perceptions, cognition, identification, and meaning would follow each other in an orderly way. But when we consider how many factors—physical, psychological, cultural, environmental, and experiential—have influenced the development of this process, we can appreciate that, in practice, the process is disorderly and easily fragmented. The elements tend to connect erratically, or to feed back and forth, giving rise to a deep-seated confusion that often manifests as disappointment and dissatisfaction.

It is not easy to sort through the strands of sensory impressions, cognitions, labels, characteristics, and assumptions, see where they have become confused, and straighten them out. The different aspects of mental activity are very mobile and do not always cooperate. But any effort in this direction will help us relieve deep-seated tension and blockages and brighten our prospects for a happier and more meaningful life.

Imperfect Communication

Each person has already established his specific reality according to the way he reads and relates to his own mental projections This can make communication difficult and uncertain, even when individuals share the same language and the same associations of words and meaning. Sometimes people say rapport and ease of communication is a matter of chemistry, but it seems more a matter of how closely the landscape of one person's inner mental realm accords with another's.

Since the private expression of one individual may have taken form differently, it may not match up well with that of others. There are differences of style that bring up biases and emotional reactions; there are differences of content and associations that also interfere with communication Then there are differences of opinion, which come from the projections of those involved in a discussion. The degree of these differences varies widely, on an individual basis as well as on a broader, more organized social or cultural scale.

Just as families have their own housekeeping and financial records, so individuals have their own sets of records imprinted in the mind. The patterns of this mental record-keeping may be based on the same model, but it varies from individual to individual, and even within an individual, as the pattern is repeated over time. The mind continues to elaborate on the pattern, as if it were mounting an ongoing exhibition. Different versions evolve, each with a slightly different character and style.

The mind itself becomes totally convinced by its own exhibition. Like a screen in a motion picture theater, the mind receives the projections of inner dialogues and stories. Their echoes feed back into consciousness, influencing how mind interprets perceptions. As a result, whatever we are experiencing, mind is also reading itself, sorting through memories and its treasury of associations, making its own dialogues, shaping its own features, and projecting impressions and judgments to consciousness. The mind seems to have its own style of negotiation. Like nearly everything else in our experience, these inner negotiations are not always harmonious. At the same time, there is another exchange going on. In grasping certain impressions and letting go of countless others, we are signaling the mind, "This is what I am looking for," or "That is not what I want right now."

We may not appreciate how seriously the mind views these signals, or how diligently it works to obey them. When we repeat the saying, "Be careful what you wish for, you may get it," we may be expressing some subliminal knowledge of how powerfully intention directs the energy of mind. If we could give peace to our mind and illuminate it with the light of awareness, it is possible that the jumbled flow of perceptions and thoughts could fall into a more harmonious and clearer progression.

How to Change the Pattern

For a long time, we have relied on mind to direct the body. Kum Nye teaches us that the body can also help relax the mind and stimulate its sensory capacities. The flow of feeling can relax the senses and open the heart. Each of our senses can open widely to different types of experience and bring in its own special qualities. Eyes can luxuriate in the beauty of light, the luminous manifestation of our physical reality; ears can hear tones that evoke exquisite nuances of feeling and cause vibrations to reverberate through the body; the nose can refresh the body with the fragrance of flowers and scents that recall memories of crisp autumn days. The body responds to the flow of wind and the warmth of the sun; as it relaxes, the cakras open, releasing exquisite feelings. Relieved of constricting pressures, the mind responds to deep flows of feeling and offers thoughts rich in meaning.

The practice of Kum Nye promotes deep relaxation, giving mind space to BE. From this, a new perceptual structure can grow up within the old, retaining the positive aspects of what is already there and allowing the negative ones to drop away. Perceptions become more full and coherent, and feelings are richer and more consistently pleasant. Pleasure melts deeply held tension, allowing us to enter the flow of feeling and expand it further. Our senses cooperate, gradually transmitting more beauty into our consciousness— beauty of color, shape, and proportion, beauty of sounds as yet unheard, beauty of fragrance, taste, and touch; beauty of thought, and depths of meaning that invite ecstasy and open wide our consciousness to wonder and new ways of knowing. Perceptions of this quality stimulate aesthetic vision and invite creative thoughts. Beauty perceived by consciousness feeds back to mind; nourished and satisfied, mind feeds back beauty to consciousness, weaving a tapestry of sensory bliss that transports us into the heavenly realms. Just as the siddhas experience and the Bodhisattvas enjoy, all these delights are possible through our senses.

From our present perspective, we can imagine other possibilities for experience than those the human senses can provide. We can understand that animals endowed with highly specialized sensory capacities might have a different range of experience, and Buddhist texts describe in detail the experiences of *pretas* (beings driven by unrelenting craving) and inhabitants of the various hell realms. Similarly, we have no difficulty assuming that heavenly beings have much more sensitive perceptions and are blessed with far more wonderful experiences than are possible in this, our human realm. But the scriptures also teach that great bliss can be experienced here and now, in this human body and with this human consciousness.

The deep relaxation of Kum Nye gives ease to the mind, relieving it of the busyness that ties up so much of our mental energy, and attuning it to what supports the whole of our being. Pathways to joy and meaning open; we make better wishes, and mind cooperates in bringing them into being.

18

Getting the Juice of Experience

At this very moment, eyes are seeing, ears are hearing, nose is smelling, tongue is poised to taste, and body is feeling. All this sensing is flowing to the mind in five separate streams, and mind is at work, busily tending each stream, alert for stimulation that might require instant response. Sit quietly for a few minutes and gently monitor this activity. Then question it softly, without disrupting or directing it purposely. Which of these streams is presenting itself most strongly at this moment? Is it the visual stream, or is it sounds, smells, tastes, inner bodily feelings, or tactile sensations? At the same time, the mind is also sensing, cognizing, and thinking. Are thoughts interacting with information coming in through the senses? Or are they overwhelming it and pushing it into the background?

As you gave attention to the activity of each of these sensory organs, what happened? Did you focus on the seeing, hearing, smelling, or thinking that was going on, or were you more drawn to identifying what you were seeing, hearing, smelling, or thinking? If so, did you identify the object in general, such as tree, bird-song, flower, or general type of thought, or did more specific information flash into mind?

The impulse to grasp and identify seems hard-wired into our perceptual system. The visual senses vibrate with varying intensities of light, and we instantly grasp for identification: We see a form; that form has a shape I associate with a horse. The horse is tall; the horse is brown. That is it: we see a tall brown horse. That is reality. That is what we have seen.

This grasping quality of the senses, a craving for contact and stimulation, reflects the tension that underlies our physical and mental systems. When we seek to relax, ultimately, this is the tension we need to address. Is there something stirring tension at this fundamental physical level? Is there a restlessness, a sense of hunger or dissatisfaction even here? Can that tension be relaxed, and what might be the benefits?

We might consider that we are aware of only a small fraction of the data streaming in from any one of our senses at any one time. Of all the dimensions, textures, and overtones we could be receiving, only the most superficial and forceful arise into consciousness, and even most of those pass unnoticed or are overridden by the few that catch our interest most strongly. If we are dissatisfied at a very deep level, it is possible that we are hungry for the full and rich experience that is somehow passing us by. We know from the examples of great yogic masters and sages of the past that human senses are capable of far greater intensity of feeling, but something seems to be blocking our ability to receive it.

Perception to Reality: The Frozen Pathway

For nearly everyone, recognition and meaning are tightly fused together. When we recognize a form as a flower, the meaning, flower, is instantly there. No doubt about it—this is really a flower, the flower is really there. This way of accepting perception as reality gives us much difficulty when we try to relax or to meditate. Thoughts come up, memories arise, and worries catch hold. We need to define meanings, fight down thoughts, and wrestle with awareness, all the while trying to contemplate. With these obstacles in its path, concentration unfolds along a winding road, with cliffs and hairpin turns. Instructions nag at the back of the mind, adding still more distractions. "I need to make my mind peaceful," "I need to let go of thoughts,"—and on and on and on. With words and dialogues cycling though our mind, it can take a long time for meditation to develop. Few people today have undergone the kind of preparation that would ensure steady progress.

So practitioners concentrate, and may get some benefit from their practice. But in trying to understand their experience, they reflexively reach for the meaning. This makes them dependent upon the recognizer, the identifier, the aspect of mind that serves as the agent of the self by labeling perceptions and assigning meanings. Once we allow ourselves to be involved with such agents, our access to the experience is effectively cut off. From that point on, we are subject to their interpretations and demands. Messages flow from thoughts to recognizer back to thoughts and again to the recognizer. Thoughts carry the messages—"You should not have thoughts, you should not be thinking about this or that, you should focus, you should concentrate." So the recognizer says "Yes, I get it. I understand. I have to do that." This kind of mental activity disrupts the development of meditation.

Language: A Mixed Blessing

Language, our primary source for communicating meaning and perhaps our proudest achievement as human beings, is a central factor in this problem. Fundamentally, language is sound that has been shaped into words. Words refer to something, such as an object of some kind, or a person, or perhaps something more abstract, such as an idea, concept, or a philosophy. Everything is already specified and labeled, and everyone who speaks English knows what the labels mean. "Tree" means "tree;" we do not mistake "tree" for something else, unless we did not hear the word properly. The word book connects immediately with the meaning of book, and the word chair with the meaning of chair. We also have words for types of experience: a certain feeling is good, while another is bad. This is unhappiness, that is joy; this is envy, this is hatred, this is compassion, this is love.

An object appears; we say its name, and the instant the name is pronounced the meaning is there. Then the meaning takes on the force of law—we cannot dismiss what that word means. Whoever first taught us the meaning of "book," that meaning becomes our reality, and we are loyal to it. There is no other name for this object but book; every other name is excluded.

The meaning of sounds can have a powerful impact on us, as when someone says, "I love you." Or perhaps it has a very different impact, if we are told, "You are a thief." We may protest, "I don't believe that." But "that" is a word, and we tend to believe what "that" is pointing to. Maybe these words mean nothing—they may have nothing to do with reality. But we tend to believe them. On some level, the meaning tends to hold up despite our denial.

Everyone knows that words have powerful effects on the mind. But the words we use daily are not words that fully connect with our experience, and the meanings they carry are meanings that have been taught to us by others. What does it signify, when our living experience can only find expression in words that are borrowed from others? Who originally determined these words? And who decided what words would have what meaning? We may be able to track a word back to its linguistic source in a distant past, but can we determine what knowledge or what intelligence gave it shape and form?

We have accepted this language; we do our best to adapt it to fit our experience, as we might try to alter second-hand clothes. But the fit is not perfect: we had no hand in its design and development, and (unless we have developed some private expressions), we had no hand in determining what its words mean.

Yet as soon as there is communication, sound comes to our ears as words. Our identity immediately slips into the process, saying, "Yes, I know what that means." The identifier pronounces the meaning, perception grasps it, and recognition confirms it.

We accept this as true because we have learned the language and already know what the words mean. Recognition simply establishes and seals the meaning, as a businessman seals a deal he has already agreed to in advance. Everything is preformed; there is no need to negotiate further. Thus words become meaning, meaning becomes reality, and that reality is intimately connected to "me." Words and meaning are now so tightly fused in our minds that it may be impossible even to conceive how one could separate them. Similarly, it is difficult to separate meanings we have learned from our sense of reality, and equally difficult to separate reality from I, me, and mine: the subject that cognizes, the object that receives, and the one who possesses experience.

Pressure to affirm the reality, the appropriateness, or the rightness of our perceptions drives the process of recognizing, identifying, and labeling that keeps going on, presenting, confirming, and re-confirming that things are the way we have learned to expect them to be. At the center of all this activity is the self, represented by "I," "me," and "mine," playing its roles as subject, object, and possessor. The reality of "I" cannot be questioned, without throwing the whole picture into disarray: "I" is obviously the director and central actor, and "I" is also "me." Whatever the sound "I" gets attached to becomes our identity, our source of nourishment, our reality, what we are. Every cycle of recognition reinforces this reality, like a self-rewinding tape that endlessly repeats.

Our reliance on language tends to squeeze the essence out of experience. "I" becomes our agent; if we want to identify or interpret anything, "I" is the one who will do that for us. While the use of "I" may sound logical, because this is how we use language, what we have done is to substitute a concept for our entire embodiment. However closely we may identify with the word "I", it is not the living, breathing being who is fully in touch with the experience. Involving the concept of "I" in the process of identifying and interpreting meaning is like putting a middleman between ourselves and the manufacturer.

Since we are buying meaning from the middleman, "I", we are losing the direct connection with experience. If we have no idea of what meditation feels like and cannot compare it to something similar, we find ourselves outside the experience, wondering, "How do I do this?" and waiting for someone to instruct us. Thinking, "If I don't understand how to meditate, how can I get into it?" is much like trying to bite into an apple without having teeth—we cannot penetrate the apple's skin. We can only sit outside the experience until our agent, "I," identifies and comments on the experience. Since our agent is also ignorant of how to get into the experience, we can wait a long time with very little result. Eventually, if the thought comes up, or someone tells us, "This technique might work, try this," we may think we have finally gotten something substantial. But it is all conceptual—all retail sales, at least two steps removed from the source—and none of it connects directly with meditation. But we do not realize what has happened to distance us from the experience.

Mistaking Words for Experience

We may not realize how easily we substitute words for experience, or stop to think about how this affects our ability to touch the living quality of experience itself. When we pronounce a word, we hear its meaning; meaning gives it reality, then we hold fast to that reality. But we may not have had the experience that actualizes it and makes it part of our being. We may say, "I need to relax," but unless we know how to relax, the words alone will not do the job: They will not take us from our stressful state to a state of relaxation. If we rely on words as our vehicle, we might remain stuck in our stressful condition for a long time, not knowing how to proceed. Eventually we may experiment with doing something and perhaps get some kind of result. But we cannot get the result directly from words alone.

This is why Western translations of Buddhist terms generally fail to hold the full meaning of the original Dharma language. Everything is labeled, its meanings frozen; there is no openness for the experience of the meaning to shine through. The assumption is so quickly made and confirmed: shunyata means this, mandala means that, Dharmakaya means that. The meanings of terms central to transforming one's view are established, recognized, and affirmed.

They can now be stored in the memory cells of consciousness, from where they can be recalled again and again. The meanings may not have been integrated into one's experience; and yet, because of the power of language, those who use the words assume that they know what they mean. How could they mean anything else?

Translators may say, "I know what shunyata means. I have read the commentaries and explanations." Or, "Emptiness is just a term that has become common usage. Everyone knows it refers to shunyata." Again, this is like trying to bite an apple without having teeth. We cannot break the skin and get the juice. We have to depend on our inner agent to tell us what "emptiness" means. At best we can embellish our familiar meaning of "emptiness" with a sense of the cosmic, or try out a number of other words, with much the same result. Even when we think we are being open-minded and considering other possibilities, the weight of the familiar tends to close off a fresh and independent inquiry. And we still have not penetrated the apple's skin. There is no opening for the experience of meaning to come through. We cannot get from here to there.

How did our language come to be what it is? We might imagine that, at some point in the distant past, a team of architects prepared the map, creating definitions and designing the structure that they felt best accorded with how humans would want to communicate. These architects may have lacked understanding and vision, but they did their best with the knowledge they had, and our language has evolved from there. Now we are repeating their design; we believe that it works, but since we do not know any other way, we cannot compare it to anything else. We depend on words to communicate meaning, and we have been given the meanings, or we can expand the concept and make more meanings if we wish. We catch on to "new" concepts by relating them to older, more familiar ones, because that is how we have been taught. But the system itself does not change. No one questions whether it still works or considers how it might serve us better.

Fields of Perception

Similarly, our fields of perception—areas of consciousness where seeing, hearing, touching, fragrance, tasting, and thought give rise to feeling and cognition—are now paved over with words, meanings, and concepts that allow us only rare glimpses of what lies below. When we attempt to relax or to meditate, this conceptual pavement tends to give rise to certain kinds of messages—"I am stuck. I am not getting anywhere." "Oh, now I understand." "I need to relax more." "Oh, there is a thought—I shouldn't have thoughts." "I should empty my mind." "But I have to make sense of this. How else can I tell if I am getting anywhere?"

Encouragements, discouragements, neutral observations—all these messages may only be meaningless mind-chatter, stirred up on the surface of mind by tension or anxiety. None of them, not even the interpretations and commentaries, can touch the inner essence of relaxation and invite the joy of experience to come out. They have nothing to do with relaxation or meditation; they cannot engage meditation directly, so they cannot analyze and judge the quality of your concentration. There is no need to respond to them, follow their dialogues, or reflect on their significance. It is not important whether you are confused or not confused, or whether or not you have thoughts. As much as possible, let this entire stream of mental activity flow by without paying it any attention. Relax deeply; allow the body to be still and the mind to calm down. Then your senses can operate more clearly, and the feeling-tone can come out. Once you become familiar with how this works, you can tune in more closely to the field of perception itself.

Tuning in to the Field of Perception

An artist may carve many different kinds of animals out of ice, but they all melt down into water, just as human beings may differ in gender, size, and features, but fundamentally have much in common. Similarly, the words mind, consciousness, and thoughts have specific definitions and meanings, but from a broader perspective, they may all boil down to the same thing. Perceptions and thoughts can be viewed in much the same way. They can manifest very differently and evoke different responses, but all have energy that resonates in our being like music. Within this silent music, there is the vibrant aliveness of the field of perception. Whatever form a perception takes—intense or weak, euphoria or sadness, bright creative thoughts or dull ones, even when a perception gives rise to fear or anger—if we welcome it and treat it nicely, we can tune into its field and direct its momentum in positive ways.

Kum Nye relaxes the tension that drives the perceptual process, allowing space for fuller, more accurate perceptions to develop. Stimulations—especially negative ones—

do not hit our hearts so strongly; the sharp edges soften and blur, reducing the emotional impact and allowing us to engage the vibrant quality of the perception directly. Almost instantly, we have access to more information; we see more clearly the context of the situation, and we can respond in ways that are more genuinely helpful to self and others. With practice, relaxation calls forth concern and cooperation in place of anger or rejection, or suggests productive new courses of action in place of discouragement. If you reflect on this line of thought and practice the following exercises whenever the opportunity arises, you will free yourself of a major source of conflict, regret, and nagging dissatisfaction.

Basic: Touching Energy of Feeling

Sit quietly for a few minutes, then listen to your body. What feelings are you experiencing at this very moment? Are they feelings of happiness, sadness, or loneliness? Are they feelings of agitation or frustration? Or are they warm and joyful? Focus on the feeling, just allowing the sensations to be whatever they are, without trying to encourage or suppress them. Let go of the words; whatever names you have given to what you are feeling, let them go. Whatever thoughts about the feeling may arise, whatever reasons may come up to explain it, just let it go. These inner interpreters are not helpful, and you do not have to deal with them now. Relax more deeply into the feeling itself. If you can stay inside the feeling, just being there, without dwelling on being anything or doing anything, you may gain some valuable insight into what is meant by the essence of feeling. If you wish to incorporate this practice into your daily program, begin with sessions of ten to twenty minutes and work up to thirty minute sessions over a period of two weeks.

Developing: Working with Inner Energy of Feeling

After you have practiced with various kinds of feelings for two or more weeks, you may notice that feelings appear different on the surface, where you have words to name and describe them. But when you take out the words and get more inside the feeling itself, you may find these differences are more like varying intensities of energy. Continue to listen to your body and stay with this inner energy of feeling. Observe its intensity—is it strong or soft? If it is soft, expand and intensify it. Attune your senses to this energy; feel it in your navel, your heart, and your throat. Surrender to it as much as possible.

Advanced: Converting and Expanding Inner Energy of Feeling

Once we become familiar with the inner energy of feeling, we find that this energy is flexible and open. We can touch it any time we wish to bring up joyful feelings, and we can use it to alleviate tension and stimulate creativity.

Accomplishment comes with practice and understanding develops with experience. As we become familiar with the physical benefits of Kum Nye, we begin to appreciate the value of relaxation to your mind as well. We may begin to notice a new brightness to our perceptions and a clean, fresh clarity to your thoughts. A quality of enjoyment may begin to pervade all our actions. At this point, we can move beyond the physical application of Kum Nye and use what we have learned to tune consciousness and awareness to a higher level of well-being.

When senses open wide to experience, blissful feelings flow freely throughout the body, loosening up concepts, melting restrictions and limitations, and opening wide the field of perceptions. The body dances with space, and space with the body; all parts of our being interact joyfully, in perfect harmony. Beauty shines through our hearts, refreshing our senses and minds with feelings of love and appreciation. Words, gestures, and postures project aesthetic qualities rich in meaning, expressions of life manifesting itself.

Eventually, it may become possible to convert all kinds of experience into knowledge that can be transmitted in positive ways. When we are able to do this, life can become an ongoing celebration, free of irritation and rough places. Agitation, pressures, and negativities that have been so difficult to control in the past can be transformed into bliss. We can begin anew and develop our own curriculum for a happy, productive life. Developing this kind of knowledge is well worth the effort.

The Fallacy of Reasons

Once we understand how language works, we know that everything we have relied on as our reality—names, meaning, concepts, identity, and the polarity of self and others—has essentially been dictated to us from the time we were born. These structures are now essential to our ability to establish reality. We have learned how to build on this foundation, developing meaning through more conceptual labels as we establish new terms and identify their specific qualities and characteristics. When we begin to see where this way of thinking leads, we might well wonder how we became so committed to it.

We make such statements as, "This feeling is uncomfortable." Can a feeling be uncomfortable? Or do we mean, "We are uncomfortable?" When we go completely inside the feeling, awareness expands it further, and we touch the quality of agitation more directly. If we ask what is causing this kind of agitation, mind begins to give reasons and justifications, or perhaps goes on to review the history and the circumstances that led up to it. Finally, the story is complete: "That's why I'm agitated, that is the reason I am so angry." Reasons give us a sense of closure; the situation has not changed, but it has been explained. Often we feel better at this point. But reasons also harden our attitudes; we feel justified in our anger or resentment, but we are also more frozen into a position that can be very difficult to change.

All the reasons that come up in our mind, together with the associations and meanings supporting them, have been given to us through language. From a logical perspective, they are insubstantial—merely words and concepts that have no empirical reality. But the way we have learned to use language has given them the power to agitate us. Definitions we have learned and adopted, based on contrast and exclusion, give us the meaning we label as agitation. Once we establish the theory that this may be agitation, it is important to go into it and trace its beginning. Something is boiling inside—where is the steam? At what point does the flavor we name agitation come up? Once we can find the point where we recognize the emerging flavor of agitation, we have to catch the point where we identify our feeling as "agitation." Supposedly this feeling also goes away. How does it disappear? Where does it go? What happens to all of its characteristics and the thoughts that were streaming through the mind as it was afflicted with agitation? At what point did they fall away? Observing the arising, identification, and passing away of agitating emotions, we gain insight into how our way of naming and identifying reality works and how we might ease its hold on our consciousness.

Melting Agitation

With any agitation that arises, the mind rushes to cognize and identify with it, in order to determine the meaning of this feeling. Normally, we are caught up in the feeling and the meaning simultaneously; we find ourselves in the middle of the agitation, with only a vague sense of how it began. When it dissipates, there may be so little substance to the agitation that we may not pay much attention to how it drops away.

Whenever you feel agitated, take this opportunity to observe how this process works. Focus first on the mid-point, where you are just becoming aware that something is happening and mind is surging to identify it. Then stretch out the mid-point and divide it into a beginning, a middle, and an end. You are at the beginning, moving toward the middle of the middle—the point of recognition, where you are being introduced to the feeling of agitation. The closer you come to this point of recognition, the more it will relax and shy away. If you sustain this focus, you will never quite reach the point of identification. The agitation will have no opportunity to become attached to you; it will run its course and melt away.

Using the Energy of Negativity

Anger, frustration, confusion, and fear all look different on the surface, but all are essentially of one flavor. Any time they arise, you can melt them down and use the essence of their energy. At first, the shape is there—the recognition, "I am unhappy." The seeds of all the labels, meanings, and associations are present, ready to develop and spin their sad stories in the unsuspecting mind. But if you give ease to the mind, you can melt down the shape of unhappiness and dissolve its characteristics, associations, and meanings into a single flavor. Then you can call forth a more positive recognition—such as "I am so very happy,"—and bring pleasant, even blissful feelings into your fields of perception. In a few short minutes, through the alchemy of Kum Nye, mind can be freed from words that identify and cause pain, from internal dialogues that give reasons and justifications, and from the emotional impact of past associations. Only the essence of their energy remains; purified of negativity, it goes into deepening and transformation, and the whole environment of the experience changes. When you compare the end result of this exercise with how you began, the value and power of this practice becomes obvious.

Give Ease to Body, Mind, and Senses

So give ease to your mind, your senses, your body, your being. Let your practice become one of "easening," allowing a feeling tone so complete, so full of balance and joy that it permeates body, mind, and senses and merges them into a unified field of being. Give ease so deep and vast that it dissolves all boundaries, passing beyond top, bottom, inside, and outside to completely fill all space, vast as the sky, beyond imagination. Give ease until the nature of Kum Nye is fully realized in your being, until there is no separation between being and Kum Nye. No longer identified with emotionality, anger, and pain, you become the experience of Kum Nye, and the blessings of Kum Nye shine through your embodiment. These are blessings we can express and share; these are blessings we can cultivate with compassion for all beings.

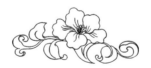

Chart of the Six Senses

English	Sanskrit	Tibetan
Six senses		
Eye	cakṣu	mig
Ear	śrota	rna ba
Nose	ghrāṇa	sna
Tongue	jihva	lce
Body	kāya	lus
Mind	manas	yid
Object-fields of the six senses		
Visible form	rūpa	gzugs
Sounds	śabha	sgra
Smells	gandha	dri
Tastes	rasa	ro
Feeling	sprasṭa	reg bya
Mental events	dharma	chos

Part Four

Massaging Mind

It is important that we enjoy our lives. But the "highs" of excitement or a few moments of pleasure make little difference in the general feeling-tones that we carry with us from day to day. The enjoyment we need is joy that flows through us like a deep current, supporting us through all manner of experience. It is the juice, the rich nectar of life itself, the source of meaning and all positive qualities. This is the kind of enjoyment that Kum Nye can provide.

In practicing Kum Nye, we aim to balance the need for guidance with the openness necessary to accumulate feelings of joy and bliss, without instructing or commanding ourselves intellectually. Any conceptual activity restricts the free flow of feeling. Fixating on following instructions precisely, or thinking about what should be happening activates the intellect; our efforts become mechanical, and we push for some result. Then the mind grows tense, constricting awareness and squeezing the juice out of the feeling before it can develop.

Since everything the intellect touches—awareness, inspections, and attitudes—is likely to stimulate tension, it is essential to ease up on ourselves. Some instruction is necessary to establish a setting for our practice, but when we are swimming in the feeling, we do not need this kind of intellectual guidance. Relax and enjoy the experience; do not hold fast to instructions or strain to follow them exactly.

19

Exercises for the Mind

Many people today would agree that they need more space in their lives. Yet space is everywhere, behind, around, and inside all of physical reality. Boundless in extent, space is all-embracing and endlessly flexible. It flows through all our reality, allowing colors and densities to manifest as forms, to which we give names. This shape is a chair; this one is a horse, this one is a car. This shape is a tree, this shape a man, a woman, a child. These shapes are fruits and vegetables; these shapes are clouds, fog, water, earth, and fire. All shapes manifest in space—in our physical space, as forms we can touch, or in our mental space, as ideas and images that can awaken feelings of love, intense passion, repulsion, or fear.

We say that physical forms come out or appear—from where? Supposedly space. We say that an idea or thought came to us—from where? Supposedly from nowhere—from

"out of the blue," that is to say, from space. We say perceptions "come to us," and in recognizing them, they become
objects of I, the perceiver, who can then watch them, do
something to or with them, or ignore them. Because the
object is perceived, the subject, the perceiver, can now
become the agent for something to happen. We might say
that the object has caused the subject to exist or to respond
in some way. But it also seems that space plays an important
role. Would there be an object without space? Without an
object to stimulate perception, would there be a subject?

This subject-object way of seeing, thinking, and acting
is known in Buddhism as relative or conventional truth
(samvritya-satya). This is our everyday truth, the truth by
which we operate in daily life. It is reality as perceived by
our senses and identified and affirmed through the activity
of the mind.

Some Buddhist texts explain that objects do not exist
in the way we perceive them. They go on to explain that
what we perceive as objects are manifestations of mind,
perceived through the activity of mind-experiencing. Since
mind itself has characteristics that affect how we identify
and interpret sensory activity, it follows that our sense of
reality is conditioned by the way the mind is trained to
operate. Consequently, the course of our human destiny—
the results of how we perceive and act on our perceptions—
depends upon the mind.

Mind-Consciousness

While consciousness is a complex and controversial topic, here we refer to the faculty of mind that cognizes perceptions and sets the stage for perceptions to be named and judged. We sense its operation in the feelings that come up in the course of our daily experience. We say "this feels good," or "this feels bad," according to how we have learned to name the sensations it evokes.

Mind, consciousness, and senses seem closely interrelated, like members of the same family. Without mind, would consciousness arise? And without consciousness to cognize perceptions, would we be able to experience thoughts and feelings? Since the nature of mind and its role in the perceptual process is in itself an important area of study, advanced practitioners may want to explore it in greater depth than is possible here. Western and Buddhist psychological traditions have different interpretations, and even Buddhist texts use different terms and explanations

Pressures of Polarity

Polarity—the way we use contrast to identify objects and arrive at the meaning of concepts—is deeply woven into our language and embedded in the structures of our minds. We do not know exactly when humans began to perceive self and other and respond from a fundamentally dualistic perspective, but our reliance on this way of perceiving has played a strong role in our cultural development. For millennia, this dualistic view has been reinforced through language and expressed in art and other cultural manifestations. We continue to operate from a subject/object perspective, which conditions how we think, feel, and act. It is now difficult even to conceive of another way of being.

As a result, we are thoroughly entangled in the webs that polarity has woven into our consciousness. These webs are dense and tight, leaving us little space for being. As our senses perceive, consciousness cognizes, and mind responds, the energy and data transmitted—feeling tones, sensations, associations, and identifications—all have to be processed in the way that the dualistic mind can comprehend. Until they are named, grasped, and judged, until we assess how to view and use them, how can we make sense of our experience? Everything has to be molded into a conceptual structure that we can understand, whether or not it accurately reflects the reality of the experience itself.

How accurately does a polarized and concept-bound mind reflect reality? If mind were operating somewhat like a computer, it would instantly scan stored memories and associations, then feed it into a program that would sort data into the categories desired by the operator. If mind is considered to be the operator, the information would have to be arranged and presented in a way that the mind could understand and interpret it.

This might be problematic, for mind's rush to grasp and interpret leaves little opportunity for clear cognition or for savoring the taste of experience. Data does not always present itself in a way that the mind can readily comprehend, and mind does not always grasp the data accurately. Yet signals continue to flash back and forth from senses to mind, crowding mind and nerves with innumerable messages urging for interpretation and response. Pressures increase, generating fresh flows of perceptions, trains of thought, and dialogues that merge with incoming data and fragment it with additional layers of impressions, perceptions, and associations. The potential for confusion is great: Signals from different sources can jam or override others, and messages tend to get mixed up or misdirected. The relentless bombardment of data overloads our body systems (nadi), blocking the flow of energy through our cakras and stressing body and mind.

Mind, now serving as interpreter, grasps for meaning—but that meaning is bonded to concepts we have learned from others, and it does not always fit well with the present situation or even with our own feelings. We may feel conflicted, intruded upon from within and without, and have no way to relieve these pressures. From time to time, our soul cries out for space: a place of calm and openness, where we can sort out the confusion, allow meaning to emerge from the heart of our being, and experience clear thoughts and positive feelings.

We can urge our minds to calm down, and we can ask our bodies to relax; we can tell our hearts that we want to feel happy and have good feelings. But how can minds bonded to conceptual meanings communicate these meanings to muscles, nerves, and senses? And how can our hearts and senses communicate their distress accurately to the concept-bound mind? Mind, body, and senses suffer each in its own realm; the pain of one affects them all, yet reso-

143

lution escapes us. On a deep level, we seem to have forgotten how to communicate with our own bodies and senses.

The kind of training that would foster good communication between mind, body, and senses is not well known or appreciated in the West. Children are encouraged to be physically active in sports and participate in physical education classes, but they are rarely taught how to exercise their sensory faculties to steady emotional energy with deep currents of feeling. Lacking this balance, exercises intended to relieve tension may only perpetuate the patterns that overload our systems and lead to burnout and apathy. Viewing body and mind as separate, the West tends to assign knowledge to the realm of the intellect, and little attention is given to the body's role as a living repository of knowledge.

For our health and happiness, it is essential that we learn ways of relaxing that bring ease to the mind and communicate directly with body and senses. We can do this through tuning the breath and energizing the senses, listening for their feeling tones, and looking to our experience for meaning instead of relying exclusively on words and interpretations. Sensations and feelings have an immediacy and freshness that can bring our experience alive in ways we cannot now imagine. Awareness smooths out the flow of perceptions and lessens the grasping quality inherent in perceiving and interpreting experience. Relaxation gives us the inner space we need for feelings to arise and flow throughout the body, and meditation engages this flow of feeling and expands and deepens it. This is the priceless value of Kum Nye: It integrates the energies of body, senses, and mind with the transformative power of awareness, turning all aspects of our embodiment toward universal benefit.

If we make Kum Nye our own by applying it in all we do, it becomes our constant companion, our source of creativity and interest, and our protection against negativity and discouragement without and within. With this protection, we do not need to regard selfishness, greed, pride, and other hurtful qualities as enemies—we can convert them into allies and turn their powerful energy into more positive expressions. Eventually, we may come to view all of experience as nothing other than mind, feelings, and mental events. As our practice develops, we can take even the strongest emotions of desire, passion, anger, and hate, place them on our meditation cushion, and melt them down into the nectar of pure experience. Knowing this is possible, we may be able to transform the most troubling manifestations of negative energy into supports for peace, joy, and spiritual health—perhaps even into expressions of compassion and holiness.

20

Orienting Mind to Joy

*I*n the Buddha's time, the Arhat Shariputra asked a long-haired ascetic what he expected to gain from his practice of severe and painful hardships. The ascetic responded that he undertook these hardships to ensure rebirth in the heaven realms, where he would be free of human miseries and enjoy a blissful existence for thousands of years. Hearing this, Brahma, lord of the highest heaven, appeared before them and said, "This earth is a paradise also. I see no problems here." To resolve the question, Shariputra brought them before the Buddha, who confirmed that Brahma was correct: This earth, this Jambudvipa, was very like the heaven realms.

Then, through the power of his meditation, the Buddha enabled the ascetic and all the monks and nuns assembled there to experience this world as seen by the Enlightened Ones. By this act, the Buddha demonstrated that beauty manifests not only in the world outside, but also inside, in our own senses and perceptions. With the right orientation of mind and senses, we can experience our present existence as a perfect field of enlightenment.

This teaching indicates that our human faculties have wondrous qualities that can transform the pressures and frustrations of ordinary existence into the bliss of the heaven realms here and now. Our body is our vehicle, and our sensory faculties can open windows to a paradise of unimaginable beauty. If we can learn how to relax, before our minds become agitated and our perceptions bombarded and overwhelmed, we can bring out the hidden qualities of our senses and appreciate their nuances and textures. If we cultivate our own inner treasures, they will reward us with bliss, joy, and happiness. Wherever we go, we can dwell serene and content, nourished by pleasure and satisfied by meaningful intimacy with ourselves, others, and the environment we inhabit.

Now, something is always wrong. However well off we are, however healthy and blessed with opportunity, some unpleasantness or problem is likely to disrupt our happiness and well-being. Our critical, judgmental minds never let us rest, and our senses are wrung dry, more attuned to pain than to pleasure. Yet if we can make our minds and senses happy, they can reveal their secret qualities and brighten our lives with creative thoughts and contentment. Relaxed and energized, they will nourish us with the full juice of experience and remind us continually of the joy of being alive.

Embodiment of Beauty

Many of us have difficulty seeing ourselves as a radiant and vital embodiment of beauty, capable of wonderful sensations, fine qualities, and inspiring thoughts. If you have this problem, or if you actively dislike any aspect of your being, Kum Nye practice can help you transform these feelings and learn to be a good friend to yourself. Then you can release these blockages, clearing the way for the senses to nourish your heart with love and joy. The senses are responsive, able to generate exquisitely beautiful feelings, but to receive their blessings, it is necessary to open pathways now constricted by confusion and stress and clogged by repressed anger and self-hatred. Kum Nye can bring light into the darkened places of heart and mind, warming and refreshing them with feelings that heal and revitalize our being.

What Kum Nye Teaches

Kum Nye exercises teach us how to smooth the jagged energies of body and mind. Using massage, postures, and movement, we can awaken blissful feelings within body and senses that can open our energy centers (cakras) and relieve the pressure of conflicting meanings and interpretations. The energy released can be so exhilarating that we may feel a sense of empowerment and momentum. We may be convinced that we are getting somewhere or even breaking through to a higher level of vision and accomplishment. But Kum Nye helps us understand that these assumptions are merely extensions of concepts we have learned. Arising from the mind's way of intellectualizing experience, they have no value in themselves. Holding on to this interpretation, giving it a false reality, will limit the benefits of our practice.

In the practice of Kum Nye, interpretations have no place or significance. Kum Nye frees us from conceptual thoughts and the need to relate experience to notions of "to" and "from." This freedom is necessary for meditation to yield its benefits and open the path to enlightenment. If we lack this understanding, interpretations will continue to thicken the conceptual webs of mind. Eventually there may be no way to release blockages and stimulate the flow of energy; the mind may become dark and the body more numb, and practice may deteriorate into a form of denial or escapism. Possibly some practitioners might regard a dull, blank state as a high meditative experience, but eventually they may realize that they are instead stranded in a barren land.

Meditation may be a way to taste the sublime joy experienced by the Arhats of the past, the long-lived ones who subjugated the kleshas and freed themselves from the sufferings of samsara. Meditation can take us even further, to the bliss that inspired the compassion of the great Bodhisattvas and led them to dedicate themselves to the liberation of others. Ultimately, as described in the Prajnaparamita teachings, even sublime bliss is transcended, as meditation melts into the unshakable samadhi of the fully enlightened Buddhas.

Meditation founded on Prajnaparamita unfolds through practices described in the scriptures as the Thirty-Seven

Wings of Enlightenment. These begin with the four foundations of mindfulness: mindfulness of body, mindfulness of feeling, mindfulness of mind, and mindfulness of mental events. Closely related are the four great intentions: to abandon all non-virtuous actions and refrain from engaging in them in the future; to strengthen virtuous actions and not allow them to decline. These practices culminate in meditative experience based on willingness, mind, effort, and analysis—the four bases of spiritual powers. Meditative experience awakens the five spiritual faculties (confidence, sustained effort, attentive inspection, meditative insight, and appreciative effort), and develops them into the five spiritual strengths that give access to the first of the ten stages of the Bodhisattva path.

Working now for the benefit of all sentient beings, the Bodhisattva abides in joy that persists through all kinds of adversity. The great being continues to exercise the seven limbs of enlightenment (alert inspection, investigation of meaning and values, sustained effort, joy, refinement and serenity, meditative experience, and equanimity), and realizes the ten great attainments: speech, action and livelihood that clear the path to enlightenment; attentiveness and meditation that advance the practitioner along the path; the view, conception, and exertion that enable fulfillment of the path; and the accomplishment of liberation and full knowledge of liberation. Endowed with these ten great attainments, the Bodhisattva enters the profound samadhi that courses like a swift-flowing river to the complete, perfect enlightenment of a fully-awakened Buddha.

We now have a most precious opportunity: we live in this fortunate aeon, when the teachings of the Buddha can still be heard; we have a fortunate body, endowed with energy (vayu), cakras, vital organs, and circulatory and nervous systems (nadi). Our bodies are expressions of the creativity and vitality that courses through all forms of life. They are endowed with senses that allow us to experience ecstatic beauty and bliss and make it available to others who have not yet seen that this is possible. If we attune our senses to the fullness of life and bring the light of compassion and wisdom into all we do, in this present body, we can experience the delights of the heavenly realms and manifest them to others. This knowledge is rapidly fading from our world. We cannot lose this opportunity to embody it and manifest it to others.

21

Making Mind Our Friend

The pressure to identify and respond to objects gives us little space between sensing and interpretation. Sensory impressions are almost immediately identified and related to I, me, and mine in the process of arriving at meaning. While these sensory impressions have also stirred up feeling tones, there is little opportunity for these feelings to be experienced as what they are: direct responses to sensory stimulation. They go directly to I, me, and mine, where they bond to our sense of self-identity.

Whatever feeling strongly impacts the I or shakes its security increases the pressure urging us to grasp for meaning and response. We are told not to "take things personally," yet when strong emotions come up, increasing the pressure to respond, we cannot always heed this advice. On the other hand, social and cultural restrictions have instilled deep inhibitions that can limit our ability to express strong emotions, so we may have no acceptable outlet for releasing them. We have no choice—we have to cope; we have to deal with what life hands us. Our bodies, minds, and senses suffer from years of "stuffing it," and we carry the knots of tensions that lie too deep for physical exercise to release.

While we may fear pressures imposed on us by others, we are even more vulnerable to our inner demons—the deep anxieties and self-doubts that intrude into our lives and undermine confidence in our value and worth. Our perceptual process, and the language we use for expression, leads us to identify ourselves with whatever feelings of worry or guilt these demons produce. The thoughts that these feelings produce can be sharp and frightening—"I'm not worth very much," "No one wants me or cares." Until we are able to recognize and separate ourselves from such thoughts, these pressures will remain with us to a greater or lesser extent, ready to surface under the right conditions.

The most fundamental of pressures lies at the very basis of what we must believe: that at some level, we have some control, that I, my central coordinator, is fulfilling the role it has been trained to play, even if that role involves frustration and pain. We see this in the strength (and sometimes the irrationality) of our responses whenever the ego is challenged or threatened. Statements we might make—"I'm not good at this job," "I'm not a good parent," or "I don't know very much about that,"—are much more difficult to accept if they are pronounced by others.

Pressures restrained tend to harden over time. Since they are widely shared, they may come to seem normal in the uncertain, rapidly changing conditions that characterize our lives today. Yet the cumulative effects of this pressure can be devastating. The lack of enjoyment and pleasure in daily life drives many people to seek ever more intense, even dangerous forms of excitement and experience deeper lows when the excitement fades. While they may look self-assured from the outside, inside they may feel restless, unable to accommodate joy, unable to enjoy their own sense of being.

Even a little experience with Kum Nye can show us that we do not have to endure pressures that are squeezing us internally and externally. Our bodies and minds are rich fields of opportunity, our foundation for cultivating a productive and happy way of life. Although we have neglected these precious resources for a long time, it is not too late to begin to use our bodies, minds, and senses more wisely, to enjoy our journey through life more fully and inspire others as well. Perhaps we have not realized that we have the ability to use our treasures in better ways; perhaps we feel it is somehow selfish to give ourselves the kind of caring attention we would extend more readily to parents, children, or others we love—even to strangers in need. But if we wish to help others, it is vitally important that we work from a sound and balanced foundation—our own bodies, minds, and senses. To begin this journey, all we need is a willing mind and an open heart.

Making Mind Our Companion

Somehow, we are manifesting in this physical form, but

we do not know how feelings come up, or how the atoms, particles, and electrons that make up our bodies behave. In many ways we are a mystery to ourselves. Yet we know that mind shows us all manner of sensations; it spins very good stories, and its presentations are vividly detailed with impressions, background information, and projections of future possibilities.

If we can free the mind of the doubts, worries, and game-playing dialogues that pressure and distract it, mind can provide us a much happier way to be. Kum Nye practice reveals the lightness of feeling that flows through all our mental activity. It invites us to enter the momentum of feeling itself, and enjoy the games of mind from a more detached perspective. Once we are not trapped in the playing fields of mind, we can use mind's talents more productively to assure ourselves of a better journey and experience intimacy with our own being. This is how we can be good companions to ourselves.

Touching the Positive Energy of Thought

Language is an imperfect tool for figuring out the nature of mind and thought. Ideas and philosophical systems may provide us theories, meanings, and interpretations that stimulate our interest, but ultimately, the usefulness of these tools is confined to the conceptual realm. In themselves, they cannot penetrate the inner workings of mind, and we may follow them a long way without tasting the flavor of meditation.

Relaxation allows mind and thoughts to reveal themselves more directly. When we are quiet, we can sense that besides the inner dialogues that come and go, mind has a kind of "beingness" quality that is silent, yet complete in itself. Nothing is missing, nothing needs interpreting. Simply resting, allowing ourselves to be directly in the calmness, we can expand this silent field of mind and touch thoughts more intimately.

To begin this exercise, make yourself comfortable in a straight-backed chair, or sit on a cushion in the seven gestures or half-lotus posture. Allow mind and body to become quiet. Let go of internal dialogues, "reminders," and other kinds of mental noise. There is no need for instructions, no need to remember, no need to monitor what is happening. Thoughts may keep cycling on, but if you pay them no attention, they will fade into the background, as if they were part of a radio program you have no interest in, but have forgotten to turn off. Let go also of the urge to understand or interpret; follow the sense of feeling as it arises, and let it reveal what the present is offering.

Whatever comes up, just let it be. Allow the petals of the senses to unfold, layer by layer, until the light of awareness begins to shine through. Relax completely; loosen the jaw muscles, the shoulders, the chest, and the abdomen, and let everything fall into the right place. When mind and body settle down in a relaxed, balanced way, sink more deeply into relaxation.

When you become more familiar with this sense of openness and the feelings that arise, the petals of the senses will open further; the light of awareness and the flow of feeling will relax your throat, warm your heart, and lead you more deeply into the calmness of deep relaxation. This is the way to begin to develop the experience of Kum Nye toward meditation. Start by practicing in this way for ten minutes twice a day for two to three weeks.

With practice, you will be able to enter the calmness of relaxation more regularly and deeply. Letting everything drop away, being totally open, you can touch the depths of mind. Rest in the openness as much as you can. Gradually expand your sitting time to thirty to forty minutes each day.

As your practice develops, it becomes easier to touch feelings of calmness and happiness, not only during practice sessions, but also during your daily activities. The more steady mindfulness becomes, the more you free yourself of the subtle fears accumulated through years of conditioning. You can become self-sufficient, connected with knowledge that comes from the depth of your being, able to engage all kinds of experience with confidence,.

Gradually, as mind turns more readily to the positive side of experience, thoughts become more flexible and creative, less likely to become tangled in frustration and less vulnerable to depression. Lighter and freer, mind becomes happy and supports happiness throughout your being. Sustained in turn by a healthy, balanced body, mind becomes your friend and companion, supporting you with more uplifting thoughts and pleasurable feelings. As obstacles between mind and body melt away, long-held tensions and neurotic patterns begin to fade, and senses transmit ever richer perceptions. All aspects of your being merge into an integrated whole, a complete and perfect embodiment. This mind and body marriage can be the basis for a truly interesting and exciting life.

The Knowledge We Need

Within our own embodied realm, we can find all the knowledge we need to go further. For the rest of our lives, body, senses, and mind can continue to enrich our physical and mental experience with wonderful feelings, beautiful sights and sounds, fragrances and tastes, and uplifting, creative thoughts. All the joy that body and mind can provide, all the streams of perceptions that the senses manifest become part of our life's journey. With such good companions, we are never alone, never fearful, and never impoverished and empty. We are self-sufficient and comfortable with ourselves, completely "at home" in the world. We have everything we need in abundance.

The taste of deep relaxation is convincing; it awakens an aspect of our being that is attuned to meaning and shows us where to look for more meaning. Once we have experienced this kind of wholeness, we know the way home to the core of our being, and we have the key for unlocking the treasures hidden within our own body and mind. The path to meditation opens of itself, and we become able to benefit more fully from the guidance of a qualified teacher. Fewer obstacles will arise, and those that do will be easier to overcome. A fresh, new life reveals itself us; we have a clearer view of our path, and as a vehicle, we have a new and stronger embodiment that can carry us to the most sublime spiritual attainment.

22

Beyond Kum Nye

The various schools and traditions follow different approaches to meditation. The tradition followed in Tibet relies on a gradual progression of meditation practices that develop understanding of prajna (wisdom) through the application of upaya (skillful means). This tradition was established in the eighth century by Shantarakshita, the great scholar who mastered and synthesized the major streams of the Mahayana philosophical traditions. At that time, another school active in Tibet was advocating an approach to meditation that involved "just sitting," keeping the body perfectly still and the mind silent. Later, to clarify the central importance of combining prajna and upaya, Shantarakshita's disciple Kamalashila described the gradual approach in three treatises on meditation known as Bhavanakrama. Kamalashila's presentation was successful, and the gradual approach became the model for Dharma practice in Tibet. To this day, it is followed by the Nyingma school as well as by traditions established in later centuries.

Certain masters in the later Tibetan tradition, however, considered aspects of the Nyingma teachings to be similar to the school supplanted by Kamalashila's approach, and even influenced some Nyingma followers to agree with them. But Nyingma scholars who examined the issue closely noted that similarities in expression were only superficial, and demonstrated that the Nyingma teachings were in fact faithful to the gradual system established by Shantarakshita. Since there are different approaches to meditation for different types of people, the Nyingma tradition has always embraced a wide range of approaches, while adhering to the wisdom and purpose of Shantarakshita's teaching.

Relying on the scriptures, Buddhist traditions recognize three, five, six, nine, or more yanas, vehicles or systems that lead to enlightenment. Some texts state that there are as many vehicles to realization as there are beings who seek to attain it. Others teach that ultimately there is only one vehicle, or go on to explain that once enlightenment is attained, there is no need for any vehicle, since all of them are encompassed in the vastness of Dharmakaya. Those who wish to develop more understanding of the enlightened state are encouraged to read the Mahayana Sutras, especially the "Diamond Sutra" (Vajracchedika) and other Prajnaparamita teachings that emphasize the importance of developing upaya (skill in means) as well as prajna (wisdom). This view continues to be upheld by all Tibetan Buddhist traditions.

Saraha, teacher of the great master Nagarjuna, says that unless meditators develop prajna and upaya together, they will fall into the current of subject and object and will not be able to transcend the dualistic tendencies of mind. Prajna and upaya have traditionally been viewed as the two wings to enlightenment. Since it is not possible to fly with only one wing, without upaya, we lack the key to complete success. In the Mahayana, prajna and upaya coexist; one depends upon the other, in the same way that awakened compassion (karuna) depends upon realization of shunyata. As the works of the great masters make clear, relying on both prajna and upaya enables practitioners to avoid serious obstacles as they advance through the ten stages of the Bodhisattva path.

Two Obstacles to Realization

The great meditative traditions of Tibet have long recognized two major obstacles that keep practitioners bound to samsara. One is the seduction of power and celestial pleasures, as demonstrated by the rishis, highly accomplished yogic sages. The second obstacle is meditation based on denial of everything, whether conceptual or experiential, which can lead to dullness and apathy. Practitioners who deliberately try to empty their minds of thoughts and feelings, aiming to make their minds completely blank, may encounter this obstacle. If they yield to it, they may stay in a state of blankness for a long time without making much progress. Practitioners who have not had the opportunity to receive proper instruction from a qualified master, or those who prefer to experiment on their own, are most likely to encounter these obstacles. However blissful their experience, however long they may sit with a blank mind, they are still within the realm of samsara.

Great Bliss: The Way of the Bodhisattva

The story is told of how the great yogin Milarepa saved his disciple Gampopa from becoming lost in the rarified realms of bliss. When Gampopa, already an accomplished practitioner, sought to become Milarepa's disciple, he hoped to impress Milarepa by describing how he could remain enraptured for a week at a time. But Milarepa shook his head in dismay, telling Gampopa that he had a serious problem. If he were to continue on this path, he would surely be reborn in the heaven realms. But even the heaven realms are still within samsara, where all beings are subject to death and rebirth. After experiencing bliss for many hundreds of years, Gampopa's life would end, and he would be reborn in the hell realms, where he would suffer for many lifetimes. This is why Milarepa told Gampopa, "It is very fortunate that you have found me." Following the guidance of Milarepa, Gampopa became a realized master and established the Mahamudra tradition, one of the major meditative traditions of Tibet.

Today, for those caught in the frustrations and uncertainties of samsara, spending thousands of years in the heaven realm does not seem so much of a problem. Many people regard that as a blessing and pray for it to happen to them. Accounts of the great Arhats and Bodhisattvas make it clear that meditation can indeed lead to sublimely blissful states. But according to Mahamudra, dBu-ma Chen-po, and rDzogs-pa Chen-po, the three great meditative systems of Tibet, bliss in itself is not enough to free us from the aimlessness and frustration of samsara. Bliss must be guided by Bodhicitta, the compelling impulse toward enlightenment that steadies practitioners on the path.

Finding Our Foundation

Although we are far removed from the Enlightened Ones of the past, we have the example of the great Bodhisattvas and teachings that explain their path and the ten stages (bhumis) that culminate in the enlightenment of a Buddha. The path is inherently liberating and joyful, beneficial at the beginning, middle, and end. We can have blissful experiences and a happy life, while also practicing meditation in a way that develops Bodhicitta. Just as athletes train to prepare for peak performance, we can develop the foundation that makes us candidates for enlightenment.

Kum Nye is based on mindfulness of body and mindfulness of feeling, the first two of the four foundations of mindfulness that are the traditional basis for the spiritual path. In Kum Nye, we use the senses to relax body and mind and experiment with the nature of awakened awareness. Feelings give ease to the body and make us comfortable. Ego relaxes, reassured by a sense of abundance, and we do not have to fight it. Feelings become pleasant and tangible; we can intensify them and allow them to carry us into deep relaxation.

Being relaxed in this way does not mean denial or annihilation. It is not waiting without thought for something to happen as a cat would wait for a mouse to appear, nor is it driven by a wish to escape into the bliss of the heaven realms. Rather, Kum Nye is based on full acceptance of the truth of our embodiment, our human being. It is our foundation, our meditation cushion that we can use to open sensory experience from within and introduce our consciousness to the power of beauty.

Cultivating the Foundation

At the instant a sense of beauty arises, before mind grasps it and propels it down the perceptual track toward identifying, cognizing, objectifying, and possessing, there is only a sensing, an inner response, a faint movement of feeling. In that nanosecond, we can be completely open to beauty, just as it is. That emergent sensing, that stirring of inner response, is the foundation that we can expand and build upon. Similarly, we hear music, and we like it. But instead of identifying the specifics and producing thoughts about it, let it be, just as it is, totally open. Expand it further. Whatever feeling you have, touch it, taste its flavor as if it were on the tip of your tongue or vibrating on the soft edge of your inner ear.

Before knowing comes in, before judgments such as "Isn't it wonderful" come, simply see the shining light or the beauty, or hear the sound, without fixating on it. Let the feeling open itself, merging with the senses, but not going further, not identifying, not even to the point of feeling yourself being aware. When you meditate, your perception may take on a subtle urging quality, as if it were a voice murmering, "I shouldn't do this," "I shouldn't expect anything," "I have instructions."

Do not engage these subtle thoughts. Stay with the sensing or feeling, the being of the experience, and let go of all that urges toward interpretation, expectation, inspecting or examining. This seems the way you can best begin to develop Kum Nye as a foundation for meditation. At the outset, this may not be easy to understand, but gradually you will come to appreciate how to balance within the feeling without taking the next step into cognition and activating the intellectual aspect of mind.

As soon as we engage the identifying/conceptual stage of perception, as soon as we think, "I have it," the balance is tipped: we fall into the second and third stages of perception. When we do this, we lose the being quality of the experience and the opportunity to benefit from its energy.

It is easy to slip into the second and third stages of perception because of our tendency to keep instructions running in the back of our mind—"I should not analyze. I should be open. I should not inspect anything." Shoulds and coulds are restrictive and prohibitive; they send the message, "That means I can't do anything."

The tendency for such thoughts to run subliminally through consciousness closes off openness as effectively as a shutter snap on a camera closes off light from film. Without sufficient openness, the image may not be imprinted properly. Similarly, if we do not receive the inner essence of the experience, our practice may not develop well. When we remember that relaxation is not in the realm of "to do" or "not to do," we can encourage ourselves to ease up on judging experience. The shutter on our inner camera will stay open longer, allowing the quality of feeling to imprint more strongly on our consciousness.

The more we relax our hold on I, me, and mine, the faster we can move past these difficulties and expand the feeling of awareness. But it is important to do this in a gentle, cooperative way that does not challenge the self directly. If the self feels secure, it will relax. When we realize it is not necessary to pay so much attention to "me," we can let go of this inner director and float freely within feeling, getting the juice of experience without grasping and distorting it. Awareness expands, and we gain a broader, more stable sense of openness that carries into our daily activities. As this practice develops, it leads naturally toward the meditative clarity and calmness known as shamatha.

Without trying too hard, we simply let ourselves BE. Directly embodying the treasures of sensitivity, we let them unfold into all-around abundance, not created by us, that provides what body, mind, and spirit need. Once we embody this abundance, we do not need to describe its character and quality to ourselves; we do not need the interpreters and instructors. We do not need to bargain for this property that already belongs to us.

Sharing With Others

Kum Nye opens the door to a new and happier way of life. Yet so many people today are pressured and dissatisfied, suffering from agitation and depression. Not knowing how to clarify the mind and invite positive feelings and thoughts, they have to work very hard to get even a little enjoyment, and what they do get does not satisfy them very long. What is the solution? They have no way to help themselves or others—they may not even know that there is a higher kind of satisfaction.

From time to time, we have the opportunity to see that more is possible: more happiness, more meaning, more joy. If we look this way, the heart opens and the mind becomes more clear. We see the value of teachings and practices that can help us; we understand the importance of taking care of our bodies, senses, and mind. We are already on the path to satisfaction.

Following this path, we focus on body, senses, and feelings, nourishing the mind with pleasure and training it to relax patterns that constrict and distort experience. These practices replace the insecurities and negativity inherent in the dualistic mind with a sense of worthiness, abundance, and joy. From this foundation, we can have a pleasant, satisfying life and share the benefits of our understanding with others.

If your wish to benefit others leads you more deeply into spiritual practice, you can continue to develop the four foundations of mindfulness and seek the guidance of a qualified master. If you persevere in your practice, you may eventually be prepared to benefit from the teachings of Great Madhyamaka (dBu-ma Chen-po), Mahamudra, and rDzogs-chen, the esoteric meditative traditions of Tibet.

23

Bringing Up
the Agent of Awareness

Recognizing the Agent of Perception

Sit in a comfortable, relaxed position. Close and rest your eyes for a few minutes, open them and simply observe your surroundings as openly as possible, making no effort to look at any one thing. Then look around you, allowing your eyes to rest on one object at a time. Relax the area around the eyes, soften your gaze, and be sensitive to internal movements and feelings. Let the mind be still, and if thoughts arise, let them go where they will. After five to ten minutes, what objects have caught your attention? Are they "just there," present in a neutral manner, or are you recognizing and responding to them in some way? Is your response one of attraction, disinterest, or distaste? Did the objects stimulate a chain of thought? Or did thoughts just pop up, unrelated to what you were seeing?

Before we become aware of a thought process occurring, light has entered the eye; cells of the eye have registered colors and patterns of light and messages are well underway to the visual faculties of consciousness. Instantly, consciousness cognizes these patterns, associating them with previously-learned characteristics in order to identify and label them. As the object is identified, the momentum of perception quickens, signaling attraction, repulsion, or "nothing special." This activity stimulates other centers of the mind; memories are scanned for more data, and identification solidifies. The object is now clearly present, and "I" am already determining how it relates to me. Although the perception has traveled far, it is suddenly "mine." "I" have become the one who sees, the one who recognizes. "I" am the agent, taking charge of this perception. "I" will direct it, express it in words, and determine what it means.

Making Meaning

We do not ordinarily express our perceptions by saying, "There is unhappiness," "There is anger," "There is sickness." For our perceptions to have meaning, it seems we need to relate them to ourselves in some way. Our language fills this need, supplying us with an agent— "I," a stand-in for all that makes up our bodies, senses, and minds, at once a convenient reference for our sense of self, and a word that allows the self to operate in concealment behind the scenes. But this "convenient reference" has great power. "I" and its associates "me" and "mine" have become central to our identity, and no other word in our language carries as much emotional impact. "I" embodies what is being perceived; "I" becomes the owner, the subject, the director of what is happening. If my senses are picking up unhappiness, that unhappiness must be related to "I;" if nerves and circulatory systems are agitated in a certain way, "I" must be angry. If there are feelings of sickness, then "I" must be sick." That assumption comes reflexively. Is there is any other conclusion possible? The perception and "I" are merged together; "I" and anger become one entity, bonded together and fused like images embedded in glass.

The links of perception—sensing, feeling, naming, characteristics, and recognition—are now frozen so tightly together with associations, meaning, and interpretation that we commonly view them as a single entity. When an object is present, the senses open, and almost immediately, the process acquires the agent—"I"—that takes charge and directs the response. We see a flower, and the "I" is there, commenting and judging: "What a beautiful rose! I really like it." We have seen the flower, but have we experienced its beauty? Was there an instant where we could perceive the play of light on the rose or follow its shades of color? Was there a sense of opening, of feelings rising to bear witness that beauty had truly touched us in some way?

Sound has a strong affinity for our consciousness, but how long can we stay with the music before the "I" comes in to distance us from its overtones and subtleties and tell us what we are feeling? Similarly, we smell an exquisite fragrance, and the "I" is there with its likes and dislikes, moving us out of direct contact with the fragrance itself. We taste, and the "I" steps forward to analyze and comment. Even our feelings are vulnerable to the "I." When relaxation releases deep feelings of pleasure, how long is it before the thoughts come. "I am really enjoying this?" What happens to beautiful feelings when we engage this train of thought?

Each of the senses has its own field of awareness, an openness that illuminates and gathers data in fullness and in depth. Awareness is not a matter of "being aware of" something. Awareness develops from the alert attention that perceives an object's full dimensionality—its depth, its luminosity, its significance—all at once. It allows our senses to savor the juice of experience, the sweet sense of aliveness that makes experience meaningful. But our senses are not operating at their full capacity. The speed of perception, coupled with the rapid intrusion of the "I" and its entourage of concepts are squeezing the juice out of our sensory experience. Tense and pressured, the senses do not open fully enough to benefit from the light of awareness.

Opening the Field of Awareness

Kum Nye enables us to thaw the tightly interlocked chain of perception. Before the agent "I" takes charge, there is a brief opportunity to open a space for awareness to shine through. To do this, rest the eyes lightly on the object, paying alert, yet relaxed attention. Sensitively loosen your hold on the object, relax, and soften the points of contact between senses and recognition. If you let go of the urge to label the object and pin it down with specific meanings, you may sense a feeling that comes from simply seeing— the experience of seeing that is free of labels and identifications. With practice, you can expand this feeling and open a small gap between sensing and recognition. Once the gap closes and thoughts come up, the naming process is fully formed, and it does not tend to change.

The feeling that comes up within seeing can be welcomed as an "agent of awareness," a way to hold off, however briefly, the emergence of the "I" and the subtle controlling omnipotence of the self that lies behind it. With practice, this feeling can deepen and expand, relieving the pressure that drives recognition and stimulates internal dialogues and mental agitation. Feeling thaws the frozen chain that binds sensing to the "I;" it opens space for a fundamental quality of enjoyment to arise and allows us to taste the nectar of experience freshly, free of labels and interpretations.

Just as the water in a clear pool reflects the image of moon and stars without being affected by that image, awareness can reflect perceptions to us, without our having to be affected by them. This is possible even with such sharp perceptions as anger. If we open a space between the "I" that is experiencing and the anger that is being experienced, we can experience the anger without having to take it on personally. In place of "I am angry," there can simply be anger. Similarly, we do not have to suffer from such thoughts as "I am lost," "I am hopeless," "I am totally miserable." These are only perceptions, transient, changeable, and without any real substance. We can simply observe and experience them for what they are, and then let them go.

If we know how to touch the roots of perception, before the stem comes out and sprouts buds that flower into I, me, and mine, we can direct our lives with greater flexibility and transform the nature of our interactions with others. We will no longer be compelled to respond to the agitation, frustration, or anger that pops up erratically in daily life. Before highly charged emotions take hold in our cakras and agitate our entire system, we can inject a healing calmness and protect body and mind from having to perpetuate this kind of karma.

When the senses open widely, they take on a different quality, and the sensations they transmit become fuller and more intense. Remember how quickly sensations flash through our systems, how easily they catch us unaware and push beyond our control. Kum Nye enables us to prepare a field of awareness that acts as a buffer between sensory activity and the "I" that interprets and reacts. To create that buffer, be watchful and alert, with awareness scanning like radar in all directions, because intense energy might come up at any moment.

Mindful Alertness

Through steady mindfulness, cultivate a mental environment that is as bright and open as possible, staying alert, but not tense. At first this takes continual attention; you develop it not by meditating a few hours each day, but by constantly reminding yourself to exercise this mental and sensory radar. Stay with the quality of alertness and maintain it as long as you can. Bring up energy to strengthen and extend it; feel the fullness of your energy stretching and empowering it, making it stable and strong. Later on, as your mental energy stabilizes at a higher degree of alertness, mindfulness becomes a natural state of being. This kind of mindfulness activates the latent powers of the mind; if you develop them well, you can access them whenever you wish.

This exercise can be useful whenever you need to address negative situations, yet are reluctant to think about or take care of them. It can help you redirect the energy now flowing into discomfort or guilt into positive action that relieves and empowers.

When you develop the mindful alertness Kum Nye fosters, relaxation unfolds as a natural manifestation of the mind's psychic power. You can exercise this power effectively to override negative influences. When you would like to stop agitation and ease the pain of unhappiness, you can do so; when you encounter mental obstacles, you can get past them and move on. That is the power of relaxation, the agent of awareness.

Relaxing into Awareness

Kum Nye practice can begin wherever you are. Wherever your body is located and whenever your senses are operating, you can attune your senses to relaxation. Make yourself comfortable, seated in the seven gestures posture on a cushion or chair. Relax any areas of tension, taking five to ten minutes to massage face, hands, or chest, wherever tension is most noticeable. Breathing softly through both nose and mouth, imagine your body floating effortlessly in space. Sense areas where tension remains; breathe in and fill these areas of tension with the fresh openness of space.

Relax completely, letting go any sense of identity—no I, no self, no comments, no concepts, until body and mind are calm and quiet, and feeling is all that remains. A body of feeling floating in space: joyful, warm, and friendly, healing, nourishing, and sweet.

As we release the tension of perception, description, and possession, we move further, beyond tension, beyond feeling, beyond even the faintest tones of feeling by letting feelings dissipate into awareness like clouds thinning in the sunlight and trailing off into space.

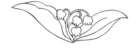

24

Surrendering to Calmness

Our tendencies to label and judge experience interfere with relaxation and disrupt efforts to meditate. These tendencies manifest in three major ways: One operates on the level of sensing, the second on the level of contact, and the third on the level of interpretation. Although these tendencies are so deeply ingrained that they are triggered by almost any stimulus, even the initial faint stirrings of sensory perception, they can be relaxed through simple but effective Kum Nye practices.

The most basic, the stage related to sensing, is a sensory readiness, a subtle feeling that poises the senses for instantaneous reaction. The senses are alert, the ears are open, the eyes are glancing around ready to record and respond, and feelings are already stirring that will point our response in a specific direction. We are ready to jump up and make a decision, although the specific reason for this readiness has not yet been recognized. Perhaps we have a sense of discomfort with how something is going on. "Something is just not right here." Even at this early point, the stage is set, and the momentum for judgment is operating. Next, at the stage of contact, the perception comes up and abruptly connects with this feeling. Then we respond instantly, "I knew it!" "I could feel it." "Now I see it!" The judgment is fully formed, ready to be elaborated and acted upon. The momentum of this process flashes instantly to the third stage, where interpretations, inner dialogues, and reasons solidify and justify the judgment. But we do not always notice this happening.

These stages of judgment, with senses poised and ready for instantaneous decisions, operate also when we attempt to relax or meditate. Thoughts associated with it are familiar: "I know I am not doing this right," or "I know I am getting better." "I am making progress." The decision is already made, the conclusion arrived at. This kind of inner dialogue indicates that we are already walking away from our meditation cushion. We are losing our foundation for relaxation.

Thoughts may be weaving their own kind of drama and spinning their own stories. Our minds may be running on a familiar track, reading their speculations, commenting on them, and rehashing the comments over and over again with slight variations, or creating dialogues in our own independent way. But all this activity is in the realm of interpretation and judgments. Mind is pointing out observations to mind, and mind is responding with opinions, also to mind. The rest of the process follows quickly in the trail of each comment, twisting quickly, like the body of a snake. When this happens, we are firmly caught up in the dialectical realm of past, present, and future, or thoughts related to I, me, or myself, involving something we need to do or understand. While we may think we are meditating, our minds are far down the tracks they know so well. We are no longer seated on our pillow.

Before meditation can progress and deepen, body and mind need to be calm and relaxed. Our senses must also cooperate, providing clearer perceptions and presenting them more gently. Now perceptions—or what we may call memories, experience, or sensory experience—just suddenly pop up, often without any encouragement or reasons. Each one presents a specific feature, as if posing before us and asking, how do I look? They invite all kinds of interpretations, and mind interprets them immediately.

Interpretations vary widely in their specifics, but they share a fundamental trait: They cognize themselves. They pop up self-contained, as if enclosed in a bubble. A characteristic of something is recognized, and an interpreter is commenting on it. Yet both the characteristic cognized and the interpreter interpreting are aspects of the same bubble. There is a subject/object relationship going on, but it is all happening within one bubble. The character becomes the interpreter—there is no other party present, no alien substance, no invited guest. The interpretations may have endless variations, but they all spring from one source. Mind reads out its own interpretation and presents it as something real. But this is mind's own private secret—it does not show us this process or how it works. The effect is much like a hologram, in which a single ray of light can illuminate a number of shapes and forms, but these forms are essentially illusions, and the light itself has no substance.

When we dream, we may have all kinds of experiences, but they are all taking place within a single bubble—all the characters, scenery, and events of the dream are unfolding within the mind. In the same way, when thoughts and perceptions come up in meditation, they may have different feeling tones, like guests arriving for a party, but they are all essentially unfolding within one mind. Light is flowing in, and the mind is reflecting different colors and shapes. Sometimes something else seems to pop up, but this is only a variation of the same process: It is still only one bubble. Mind is reading itself—there is no second interpreter. Since the process is largely hidden, the meditator may not be aware of how this works.

As long as we remain on the level of interpretations, we cannot experience the calmness necessary to engage meditation fully. Trying to meditate with the mind occupied by internal conversations is like trying to pour nectar into a cup while we are running too fast to hold the cup steady—we end up spilling most of it and cannot fully enjoy the taste that remains. As long as our interpretations and explanations are in action, reporting back to us what the concept of relaxation means, making up stories about how to do it, and assessing how well we are succeeding, we will have a hard time embodying the total relaxation.

When we understand how this process operates, it seems very simple and perfectly clear. But when we do not understand, it is very complex. We can never figure it out, no matter how intelligent we are, because the intellect has no access to its own workings. As soon as it attempts to investigate, the mind moves, and the movement changes the characteristics. A different story continues, changes again, and more stories come. We cannot touch or capture these stories with more stories; we cannot use the mind to figure out the mind. That is why it is essential to relax body, breath, and senses and open up this process from within.

Stories We Tell

If we have some insight into how thoughts and perceptions become entangled in the patterns of mind, we have knowledge that will save us much time and frustration when we wish to practice meditation. So it is helpful to reflect on how thoughts and perceptions manifest in our experience. Sitting quietly on our cushion or chair, we may think we are meditating, but in a short time, our minds may be very active, telling stories and weaving fantasies that convince and distract. We might notice these thoughts and push them away, thinking, "I'm trying to relax." In doing this we are actually disturbing the calmness of mind and disrupting the development of meditation. Or we may be focused, perhaps curious or expectant, intent on watching meditation "happen." This watchful approach is also disruptive, as if we were to touch our reflection in a clear pool of water in an effort to see our image more clearly. The more we try to touch what is there, the more we disturb the water and fragment the image. So the best way to proceed is to allow mind to become totally calm—without disturbing and without making efforts to figure out or judge what is happening. Just take a few moments to develop a general feeling for how to sit, how to breathe, and how to be, then let go of all these concepts—let go of the instructions, let go of interpretations of the instructions, and let go also of these instructions about the instructions.

How Patterns of Mind Interfere with Meditation

When we are asked to let go of instructions, it may seem as though no instructions are needed. If there is nothing to be done, what is the point of "doing meditation?" It may not be immediately apparent how to "let go" of instructions or how it is possible for instructions to obstruct relaxation or meditation. Told on the one hand that instructions and suggestions are necessary, and on the other that holding on to them is not helpful, the aspiring meditator may feel stuck in a conundrum. "So what should I do?" "Now I'm just sitting here, not doing anything. I am relaxed, I am being quiet. This must be what is meant. This must be the best way to meditate." The meditator is supposedly doing what he or she is supposed to do, but the mind is still active and searching, trying to make meaning out of what it does not understand. "The instructions say to let go of instructions, so I have done that. Now I am waiting. What happens now?"

Instructions tend to flicker through the mind like an echo of our own voice: "What should be happening?" "Am I feeling more calm?" "Am I having thoughts?" "Am I being mindful enough?" "Am I watching like I'm supposed to?" We may feel very silent, but this kind of mental noise tends to echo in the back of our minds. These mind-echoes indicate that the invisible instructor is still holding on—"I" am watching, "I" am reminding, "be aware!" This sense of watching inhibits the openness of relaxation and tightens the mind, closing off feelings of bliss. This invisible instructor is not needed, so it is better if it is not there.

Opening the Gateways to Meditation

Lacking direct access to any other way of understanding, we have to rely on instructions. But if we rely on them, we may find ourselves caught up in the games of our concept-driven minds. How can we proceed in a balanced way, when we can perceive no middle ground?

If we understand that instructions are both necessary and limited, we can work with them, aware that here also, Kum Nye can be helpful. Our practice of Kum Nye can help us loosen up tendencies to hold on tightly to concepts and expectations. It can help us notice and relax the internal "watcher" that tenses the mind, nerves, and senses and numbs our experience, and it can support the patience necessary for experience to develop. In the same way we have learned to surrender to the flow of beautiful feelings, we can surrender to the silent calm of meditation. In the openness of relaxation, nourished by the vital energies awakened by Kum Nye, the open awareness of meditation begins to develop.

Reflect on instructions ahead of time so you have some idea of how the exercise or meditation practice develops, but be mindful that individual experiences will vary, so expectations will distort or block the unfolding of meditation. Since thoughts and perceptions pop up within the field of meditation and cycle around and back and forth without going anywhere outside it, you can open them up by loosening mind and body, and relaxing as fully as possible. Allow a sense of ease to develop. Let go of all the stories and inner dialogues; let go of the interpretations. Let go even of the thought that you are observing; let go of any notion of the way to know or meditate. Even let go of instructions.

"But I don't know how to do this!"

"Let go" means whether you know or don't know, let go even the dialogue about knowing or not knowing. Words that give you a sense of knowing are not important, and instructions can only point out where to begin. When you are actually doing the exercise, depending on formal directions will obstruct your progress. When you are completely within the meditation, you know it. Then there is no need for instructions or interpretation.

Trust your experience and follow the deepening current of meditation. When feeling arises, breathe into it and let it open up. Do not fixate on it, and do not ignore it. Relax completely; relax the interpreters, relax the judgmental, thinking, dialogue-making observers, and relax the radar-like sensitivity that feeds this speedy, jumping quality. Tune it down, as if you were turning down the volume of a radio, and rest in the openness of meditation.

Completely embody calmness: let calmness itself become being. "Becoming being" means: there is no particular shape or form to direct your attention to, and no I, me, or mine to do the directing. Let mind, thought, feeling, judgments, perceptions, any awakened kind of awareness or mindfulness—all the aspects of mind that notice and identify—be completely open, without any qualities that invite interpretation. You do not need any interpreters mediating between experience and being. These labels and all their associations have no meaning here.

Practice surrendering to calmness silently by yourself for a few hours every day. If possible, extend your practice in four-week retreats several times a year. The fullness of the Kum Nye experience makes mind and senses very sensitive and tender; perceptions become smooth and clear, and the feelings that they awaken transmit sweetness and warmth throughout your being.

Rejecting nothing, accepting nothing, setting up nothing—these are the guidelines for relaxation that opens wide the gateways to meditation. There is no need to improve or fix anything; there is no need to stamp out thoughts, no need to add anything or take anything away. When there is nothing to distort the clarity of direct experience—no concepts, no sensations, and no memories, no body, no mind, no senses, not even any awareness of you yourself being— there is only being. This is the kind of experience we need.

Let Blessings Be

These instructions are offered to point out the importance of letting go of instructions, so you can crack the shell of concepts and restrictions and taste the calm, healing essence of pure experience. Even so, now that the word being has been used, because of language and the polarity it depends upon, you may get caught up into watching for whatever meaning you attach to the concept of being. As long as polarity influences your consciousness, any movement, any tickling of your perceptions, will tend to flow into the subject/object realm of dualistic mind. If you are aware of these patterns and understand how tenacious they can be, your path will be easier and more joyful. So once you have tasted some kind of flavor within relaxation or meditation, encourage yourself to persevere, without depending on concepts or any kind of instructions, resolving never to give up.

When you surrender and let go, sometimes, without any instructions and when least expected, blessings may come. To benefit from these moments, train yourself from the outset to let these blessings be, to allow space for something new and positive to develop that is truly your own. When these moments come, relax completely into the experience and let it open and expand as far as it will go. If you can do this, blessings will come more frequently; the petals of the heart will unfold, and energy will expand beyond your body, releasing the webs of restrictions, melting obstacles in your path, and clearing away from your being the shadows of emotionality and negativity.

Developing the Kum Nye Experience

Kum Nye releases the pressures of obligations and commitments that accumulate in the course of our tightly scheduled, busy lives. It gives us the key to deep relaxation, and its basic principle is clear and straightforward: Loosen up!

Loosen up all areas of tension—in the body, in the senses, in the mind. Whatever feeling tone comes out, let it be. Stay quiet and calm, and sink into the feeling. You may feel a sense of opening, as if your heart were a lotus flower just beginning to blossom.

In the mornings and evenings, set aside a specific amount of time for Kum Nye and dedicate it to your practice. Open the first petals of feeling and relax into calmness; then relax more, again let the feelings be, then relax further, sinking into them more deeply with each repetition. These are the stages of relaxation that draw in the feeling. As the first soft petals open, you can feel your heart opening more widely. You can go inside the feelings and invite healing. Let the feelings be, refraining from taking possession of them or interpreting them. Go along with the current of feeling and allow it to deepen. You can apply this way of working with feeling as you do any of the exercises in this book.

Once we become familiar with the experience of Kum Nye, and know how to surrender to calmness and inner peace, there will be no need for further instruction or guidance. Kum Nye will reveal itself naturally. The process will continue to develop and become deeper and vaster. Eventually, it will encompass all of experience, dissolving problems and obstacles, and encouraging the mind to reveal its treasures more fully. Mind itself can become a source of innovative relaxation, a mine of pleasure, vitality, and creativity that we have yet to discover. Operating within the Kum Nye experience, mind can become a continuous wellspring of positive energy, a powerful ally in transforming negative patterns and directing healing energy throughout our bodies.

The beauty of our internal understanding can expand far beyond the conceptual frame of reference, rippling out beyond the farthest reaches of imagination, where language cannot capture it, and the critical mind cannot comment. Here logic and philosophy have no place to stand. But our internal evolution can continue to unfold, expanding awareness and pointing ever more surely toward the full development of awakened mind.

Part Five

Advanced
Kum Nye Exercises

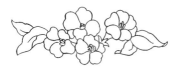

General Guidelines for Exercises

Always begin and end a session of exercises with the Seven Gestures.

Always breathe gently and evenly through both nose and mouth unless the exercise specifically directs otherwise. Pay special attention to the evenness and softness of the breath at the beginning and ending of each exercise. Do not hold your breath, but let it flow smoothly for it is the breath that touches and unlocks blockages. The breath transports the energy of the blockage into the flow of feeling.

When taking a posture or performing the movements, do not strain or force yourself, but do not hold back your full participation as best you can.

Each exercise can be practiced on at least three different levels:

- taking the physical posture or making the movement
- contacting the flow of feeling
- deepening and expanding the experiences

Each exercise can be practiced with different focuses depending on which section of this book you are engaging:

- the breath
- the senses and perception
- the mind

Group One

Integrating
Body & Mind

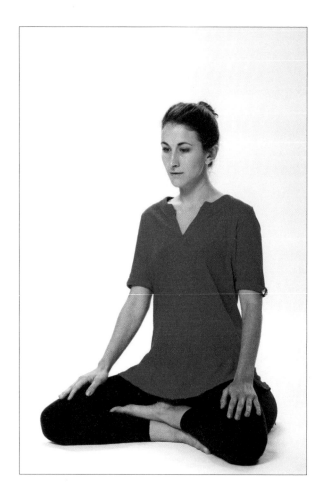

Half-Lotus Sitting Posture

Take the posture of the Seven Gestures. Sit cross-legged in the half-lotus position. Place your hands palm down upon your knees. Straighten the spine and gently pull your shoulders back. Tuck your chin in slightly. Leave the mouth slightly open. The tongue is curved back a little, lightly touching the palate behind the teeth. The eyes should be half-closed, the gaze focused toward the tip of the nose. See "Seven Gestures" in Part One.

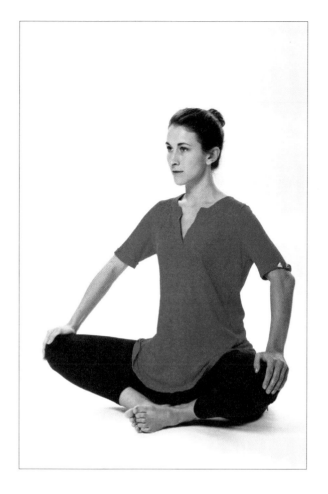

Releasing Energy

Sit half-lotus style on a cushion or on the floor. Then draw up your knees and put the soles of your feet together. Push both the knees down at the same time and hold a moment. Keep the back straight and the head straight. Release the legs and feel the energy flow in the hips and legs. Repeat three times.

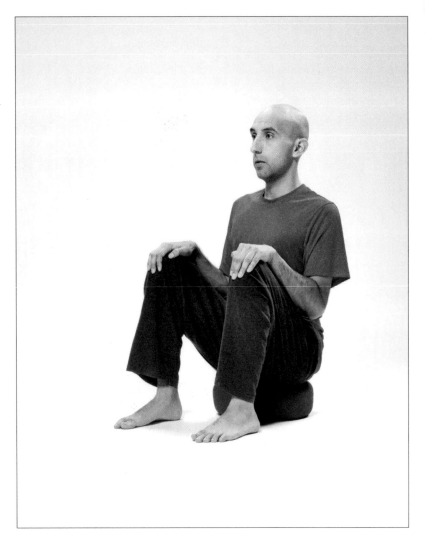

Freeing Energy - Step One

Sit on a cushion with your back straight and your chin tucked in. Bend your knees and bring them both up together but not touching. Place your palms on your knees, keeping your feet flat on the floor about one foot apart.

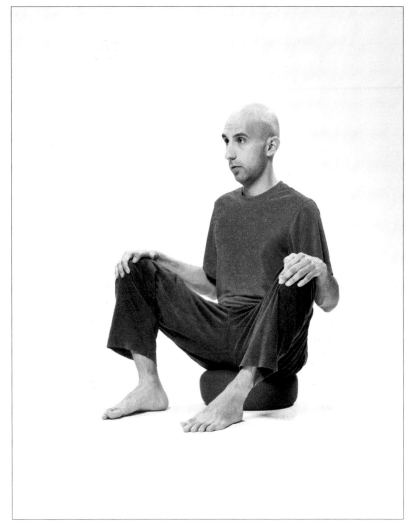

Freeing Energy - Step Two

Widely open your knees and push them both down at the same time, and hold a moment. Then bring them back together. Repeat six or nine times and then sit in the half-lotus position.

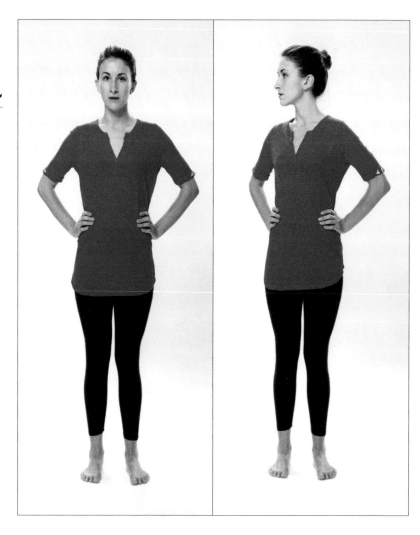

Inviting Feeling

Stand in a relaxed manner with your hands on your hips and the elbows pointed out to the sides. Twist to one side from the waist up, letting your head move with the shoulders while leaving the hips and lower body in place. Repeat three times, twisting to each side. Then relax your arms and stand completely still.

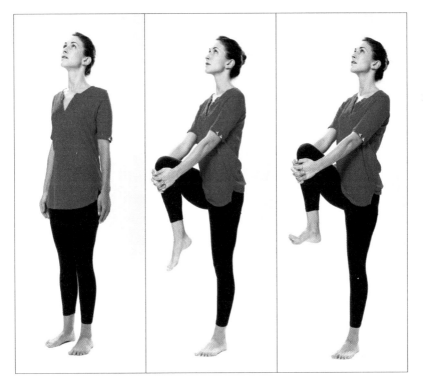

Body & Mind Balance

Stand comfortably with arms relaxed at your sides and head tilted slightly back, your eyes gazing upward. Pay attention to the energy flowing through your neck, back, and feet. Note the sensations associated with the body feeling stable and well-balanced.

Bend one knee and bring it up toward your chest slowly without losing your balance Wrap both hands around the knee and pull it toward you. Let your body rebalance naturally in this position. Notice the energy flow in the legs and the back.

While in this position, gently raise the toes of the foot and hold the position. Repeat three times on each side.

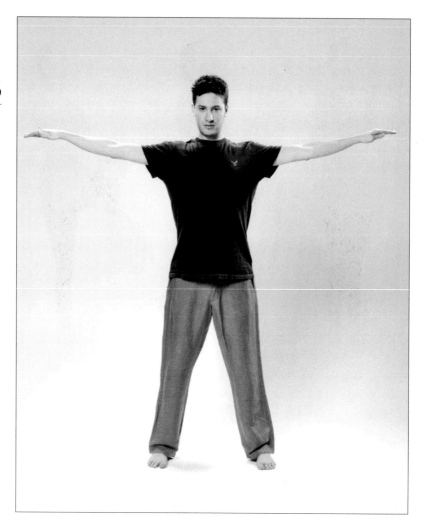

Connecting Feeling - *Step One*

Stand comfortably with your feet apart and your knees straight but not tightly locked. Tuck your chin in slightly and keep your back straight. Stretch your arms out to each side at shoulder height, the palms facing down. Gently notice the energy in your shoulders and arms, and in your legs and feet.

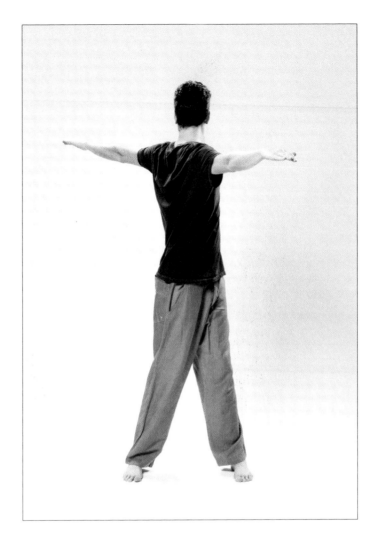

Connecting Feeling - Step Two

Keeping your feet pointed forward, twist to the left as far as you can, with your arms outstretched. Let your head move with your shoulders as you twist. Hold for a few moments and then return to center. Repeat this twist three times. Then twist to the right as far as you can. Repeat this twist three times. Then relax deeply.

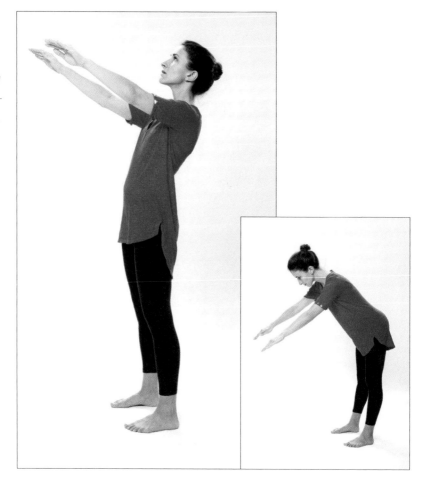

Opening the Flow - Step One

Stand with feet apart, your knees straight but not locked tightly, and your arms held out in front of you at shoulder height. Gently and slowly bend backward, arching the neck and letting the head tilt back. Then slowly bring the head forward to upright, and then continue the movement forward and down by bending at the waist.

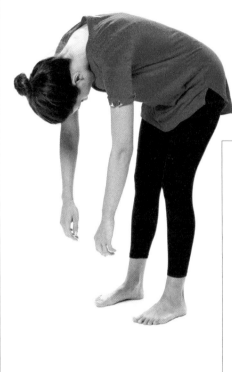
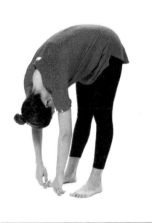

Opening the Flow - Step Two

Continue bending forward, letting your arms and head hang loosely down. Completely relax your neck and stay in this position for a few moments. Come up slowly by straightening at the waist, letting your arms and head hang loosely as the body moves toward upright. Notice the strong energies starting to flow through the body. Slowly return to an upright posture, arms at your sides, and stand completely still for a while.

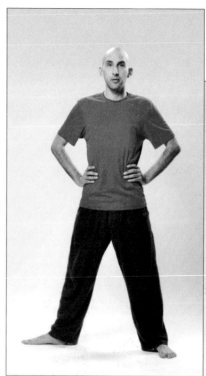
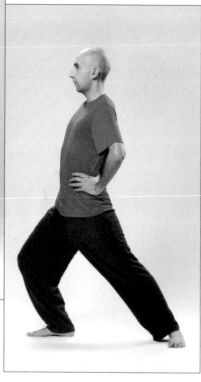

Mind & Body in Space - *Step One*

Stand comfortably with your hands on your hips and straighten your back. Point one foot forward and the other to the side about three feet away. Bend the knee on that side and twist at the hip toward that side. Leave the other leg facing forward and straight.

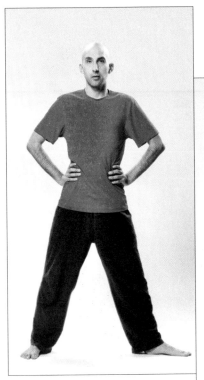

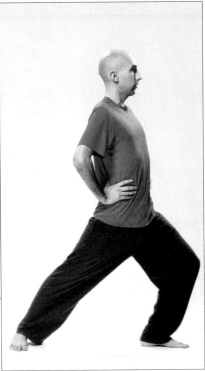

Mind & Body in Space - *Step Two*

Then return to the original position and pause a moment. Repeat this twisting motion three times on each side, each time returning to the original centered position and pausing. Pay special attention to the space through which you are moving moment by moment.

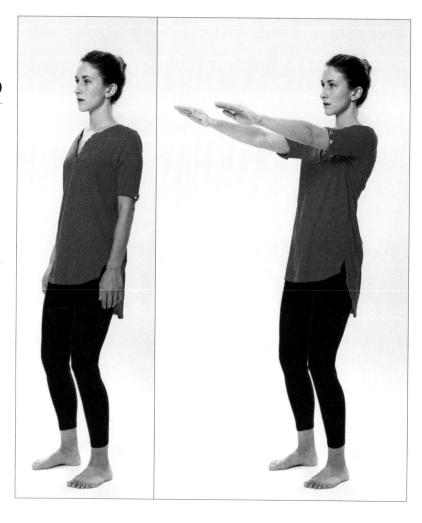

Mind & Body Touching

Stand with your feet a little apart and your arms relaxed loosely at your sides. Then slowly bend your knees, push the chest back, let your spine arch gently and open up the knees a little. Raise your arms to shoulder height and leave them extended as you move up and down three times slowly. Then relax your arms at your sides and remain in stillness.

Group Two

Embracing Space

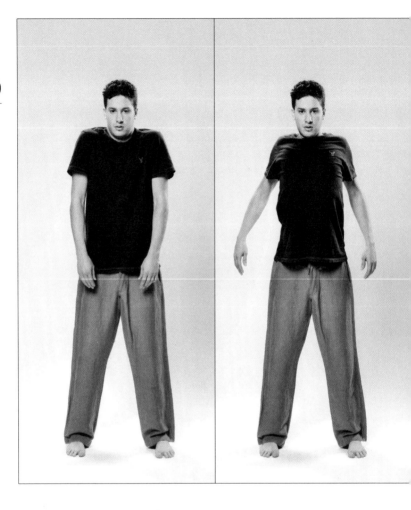

Relaxing into Space

Stand with your arms relaxed at both sides, palms facing the body. Bring both shoulders in and up and rotate together forwardly and backwardly in a circle. Pull the stomach in and tighten the abdomen, leaving the mouth open. When you stop, release the neck and loosen the chest and belly. Focus on the border where the solidity of the body meets space and gently expand that feeling a few inches outside the body and into space.

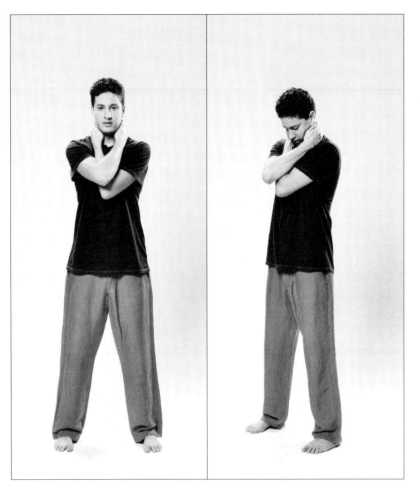

Healing Inner Space

Stand with your arms folded over your chest. The palm of the left hand is along the right side of the neck, and the palm of the right hand is along the left side of the neck. Press the chin down and close the eyes. Hold this position a little while. Then release slowly, bringing your arms back to your sides.

Releasing Solidity - *Step One*

Stand with your arms relaxed at your sides. Move the head up and down by simply bending the neck straight down and straight up. Go back and forth several times.

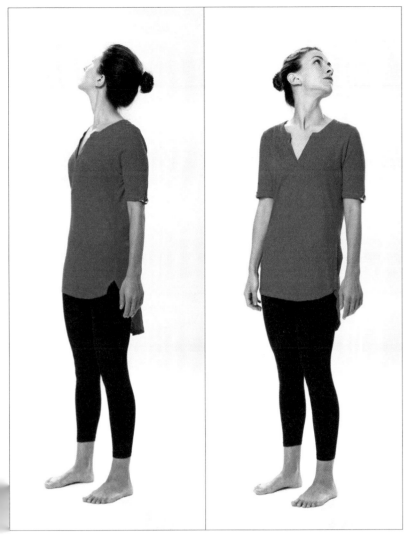

Releasing Solidity - *Step Two*

Then stretch the neck to one side and up so that you are pointing your chin at the ceiling, keeping the eyes open, and looking strongly outward. Hold a little while, and then release.

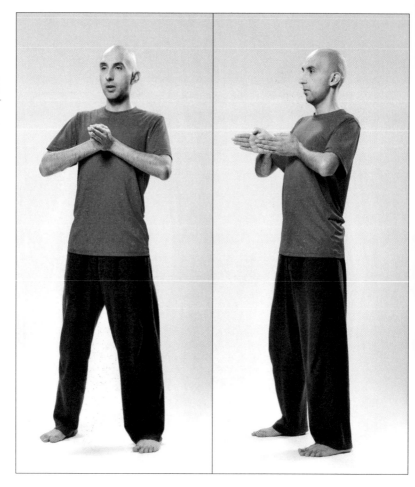

Hand Magic - *Step One*

Stand with your hands held in front of you at heart level with your elbows bent. Bring the palms of your hands together, fi ngers pointing forward. Then push one hand against the other strongly. Slide the hands back and forth over each other, gradu-ally moving faster and fast-er. When the hands feel quite warm, stop the movement and bring the hands together palm to palm, and then gently, slowly move them apart an inch or two. Then bring them together again and move them slowly apart.

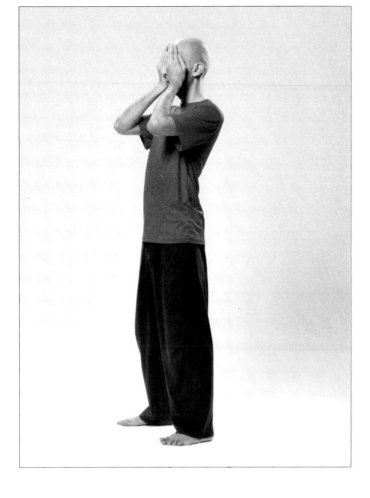

Hand Magic - Step Two

As you make these motions between your hands smaller and smaller, you may sense energy or pressure between the hands. When you can feel this sensation, place both hands over your eyes and let the energy flow into the face, releasing all the tension in your face, head, and neck.

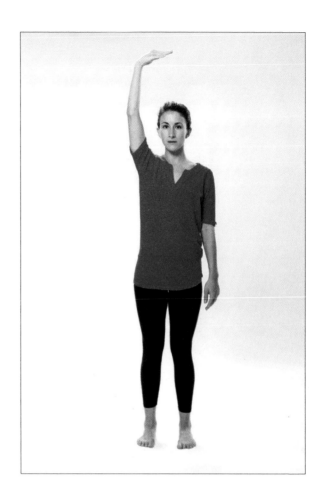

Evoking Space

Stand with one hand held above the head bent at the wrist, with the palm facing the top of your head. The other arm is relaxed at your side. Rotate your arm in a circle above the top of your head, keeping your fingers flat. Leave your mouth open. Then raise the other hand and reverse the positions. Stretch the muscles of the rib cage upward as you do these circular motions, and let the mouth remain open. After a few minutes, relax in a standing posture.

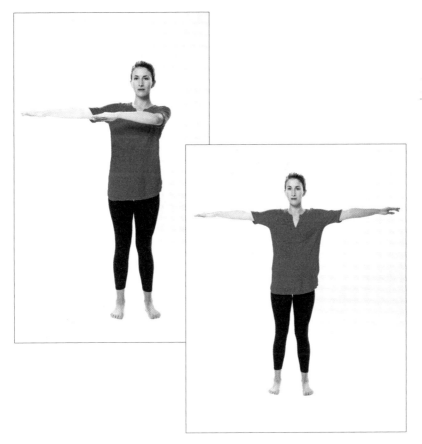

Touching the Heart of Space

Take a standing posture with your arms extended both to one side at shoulder height. Notice the space between the hands. Then move one arm back to its own side, so that you are standing with both arms out to both sides at shoulder height. Then move both arms to the other side and extend them. Again, notice the space between the hands. Finish by moving one arm back to its own side, so you are standing with both arms out to both sides. Then lower your arms and deeply relax.

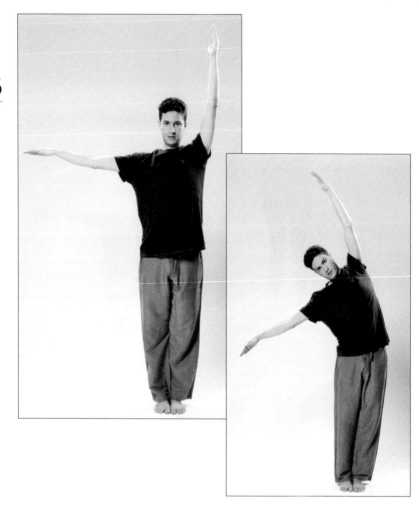

Space of Joy

Stand with your feet together. Raise one arm straight up close to the side of your head and extend the other arm out. Tilt to the side where the arm is extended, keeping your face pointing toward the front. Keep your knees straight and push energy towards your feet. Repeat on the other side.

Group Three

Stimulating
Inner Energy

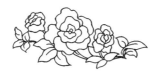

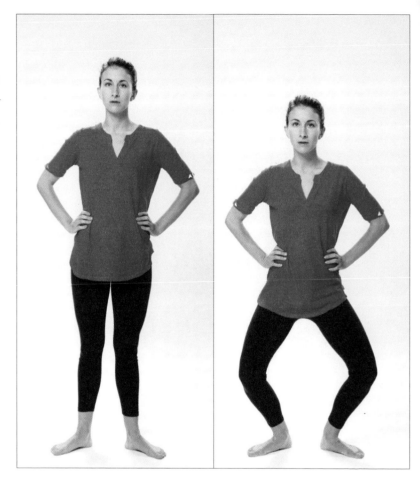

Loosening Blockages - Step One

Take a standing posture with your feet turned out and your heels about five inches apart. Bend at the knees, placing your hands on your hips, and sink down as far as you can. Hold the position until energy is moving in the lower body.

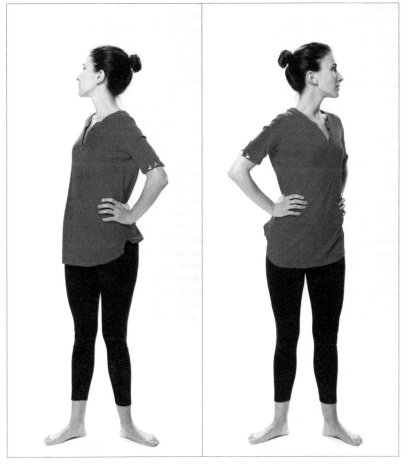

Loosening Blockages - Step Two

Come up gently to a standing position and then twist three times to each side with your hands still on your hips. Complete the exercise facing forward with hands on hips. Deeply relax the hips and shoulders and let energy move.

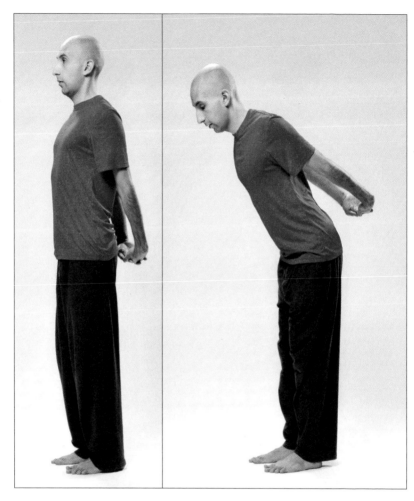

Extending Energy - Step One

Take a standing posture with your feet four inches apart. Put both hands behind your back at waist level, interweaving the fingers and extending the elbows. Bend forward at the waist, moving gently, keeping your knees straight and letting your elbows rise up.

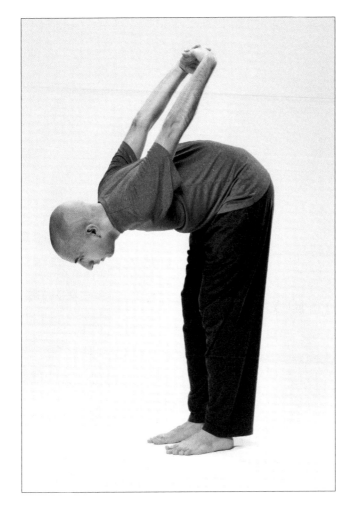

Extending Energy - Step Two

Bring your arms up higher and let the head hang down lower. Then shake your head gently from side to side. Pay attention to the sensations in the lower spine and how energy flows up the spine. Straighten up, letting your knees bend and keeping your arms behind your back until you are upright. Then relax hips, belly, and shoulders. Finally, release the arms. Pause a moment.

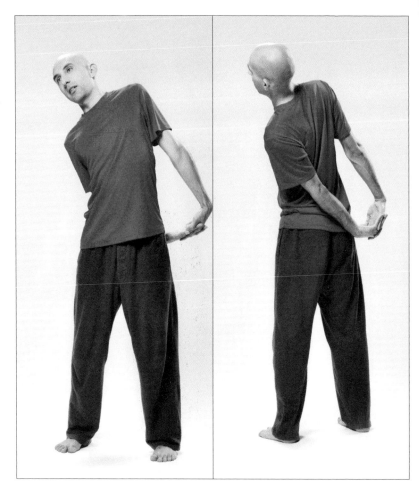

Extending Energy - Step Three

Move your feet apart eight inches. Put both hands behind your back at waist level again, interweaving the fingers and extending the elbows. Bend to one side and hold the position. Then straighten up slowly. Then bend to the other side and hold. Straighten up slowly and pause.

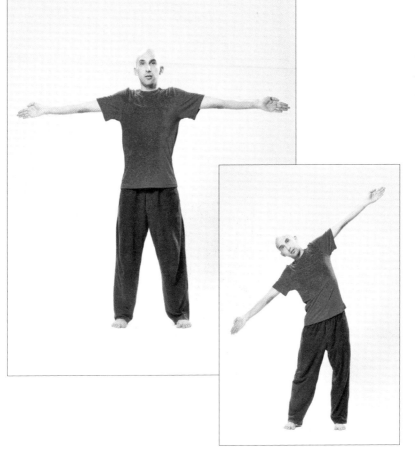

Extending Energy - Step Four

Extend your arms to shoulder height and hold your hands out with palms flat and facing outward. Bend gently to one side, with both arms extended. Return to the center. Then bend to the other side. Repeat several times. Pause for a moment.

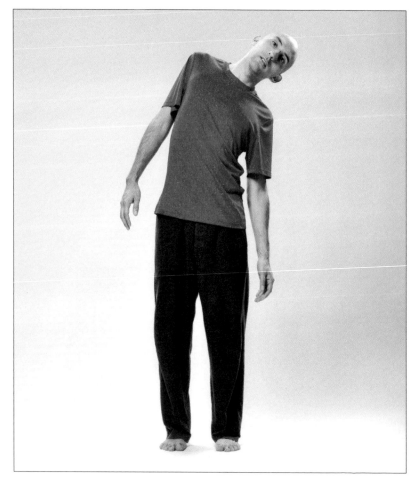

Extending Energy - Step Five

Let both arms hang loosely at your sides, completely relaxed. Bend to one side letting one shoulder move lower and the other shoulder rise up. Hold the posture a moment and then return to the center. Bend to the other side in the same way. Then return to the center and exhale deeply. Relax completely and remain in this standing posture for several minutes.

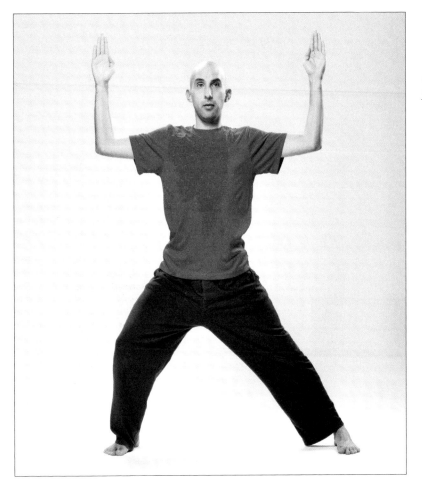

Ground of Energy

Stand with one leg to the side, bent at the knee, and the other leg to the other side, with the knee straight. Hold both hands up, elbows bent square to the ground. Keep your face forward and your palms out. Breathe deeply and relax, holding the body very still. Then switch legs and repeat. Do three times each side. Then bring your arms slowly down to your sides and stand still.

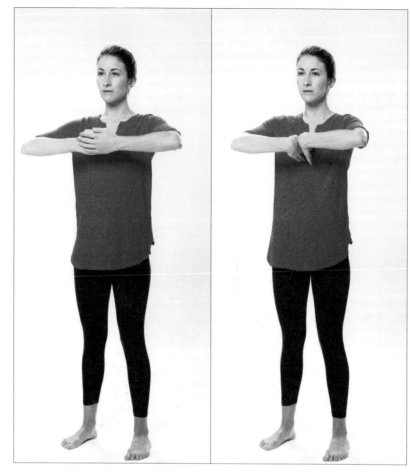

Circulating Energy - *Step One*

Stand with your arms at heart level, palms facing your chest and hands overlapped, with fingers extended. Slowly move hands apart and curve them both in towards the chest, letting the elbows move forward, and the backs of the hands touch. Hold this position. Then release the hands back to the starting position. Repeat several times. Then stretch your arms out in front of you palms down and spread the fingers widely, releasing the energy.

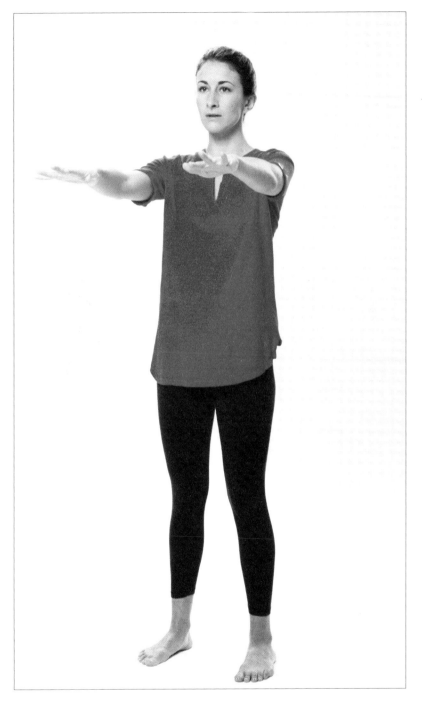

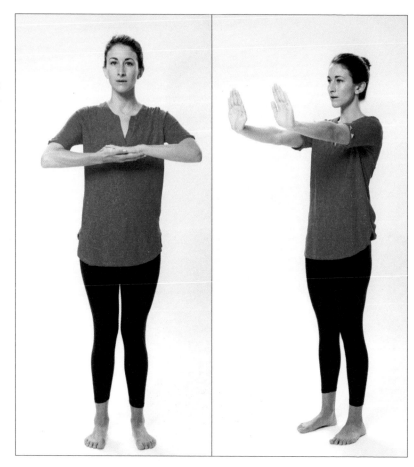

Circulating Energy - *Step Two*

Stand with your arms at heart level, one palm facing up and the other down. Bend your elbows and press down with one hand and up with the other. Reverse the hand positions and repeat the pressing. Then turn your hands out and extend your arms straight in front of you. Keeping elbows extended and palms out, move your arms in a circular motion in front of you. Turn at the waist and make circles on each side. Conclude by returning your hands to the starting position and release the energy.

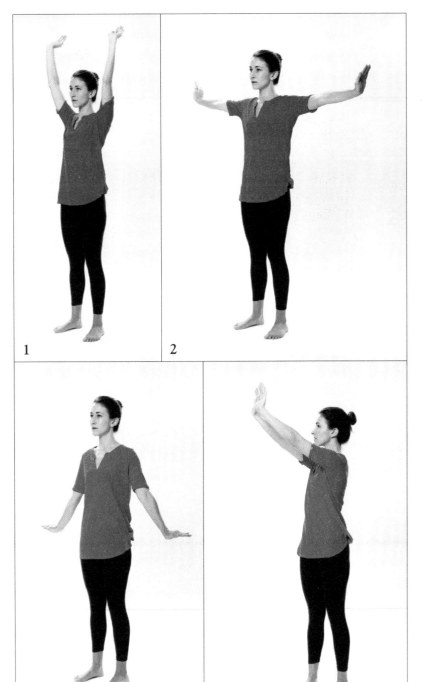

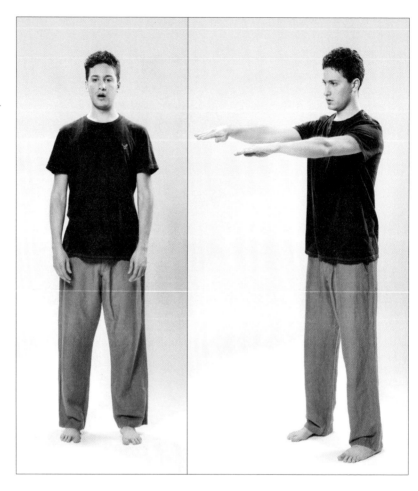

Opening Energy - Step One

Stand with hands relaxed at your sides. Take a deep breath and open the chest with HAA pronounced loudly. Then raise your arms to shoulder height and extend them in front of you. Hold this position for a moment.

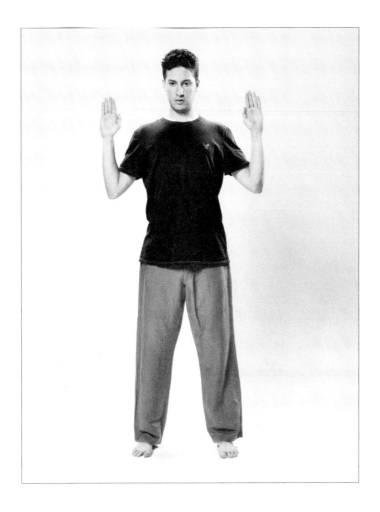

Opening Energy - *Step Two*

Then slowly pull in your arms, bending at the elbows, holding the palms outward and keeping the hands at shoulder height. As you pull in your arms, tighten the belly. Hold this position for a moment. Then loosen the belly. Repeat several times.

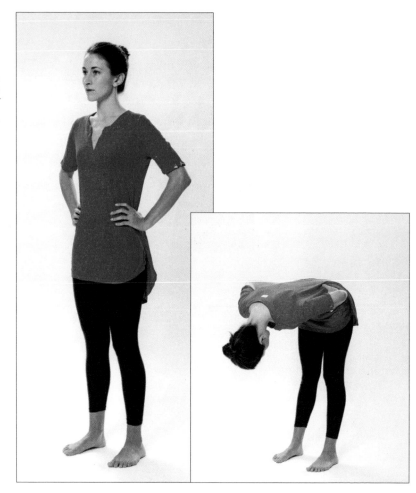

Exercising Energy - Step One

Stand with your hands on your hips and then bend at the waist and let your head hang down. Pause. Then widely open the feet and let your arms and head down gently until your hands are flat on the floor or as close to the floor as you can reach. Slowly straighten the knees so the body makes an upside down V, with legs widely apart and hands about one foot from your feet.

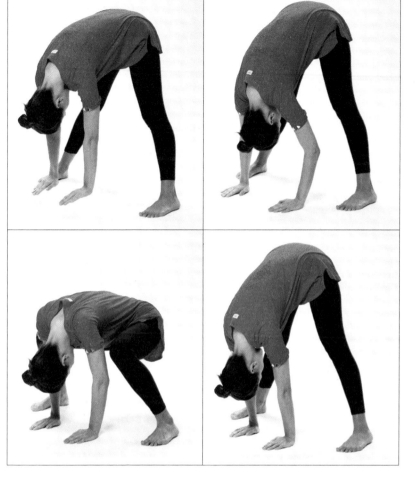

Exercising Energy - Step Two

Push your hips up and then bend at the knees to bring the hips down. Raise your hips up and down several times. Try bringing the feet closer together and raising hips up and down in the same way. Then slowly come up. Pregnant women or those with migraine should not do this exercise.

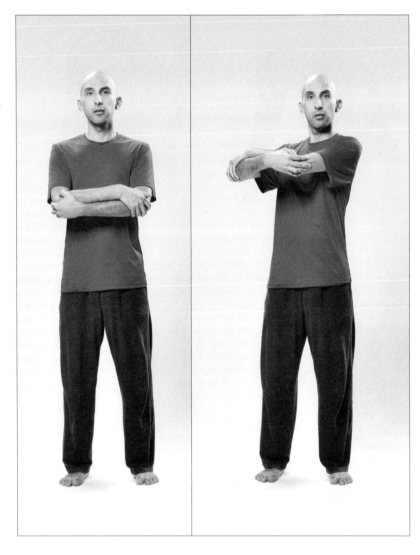

Embracing & Uplifting - Step One

Stand with your feet a little apart. Fold your hands across your chest so that your hands are grasping your elbows. Twist to one side keeping the face forward. Then twist to the other side. Repeat three times on each side.

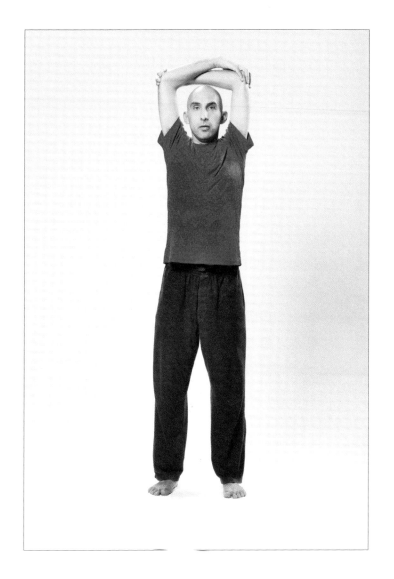

Embracing & Uplifting - Step Two

Raise your arms up and down, while leaving them folded. Repeat three times. Then release your arms down to your sides. Breathe lightly, pulling the stomach in a little. Visualize the flow of energy in your arms, hands, and fingers.

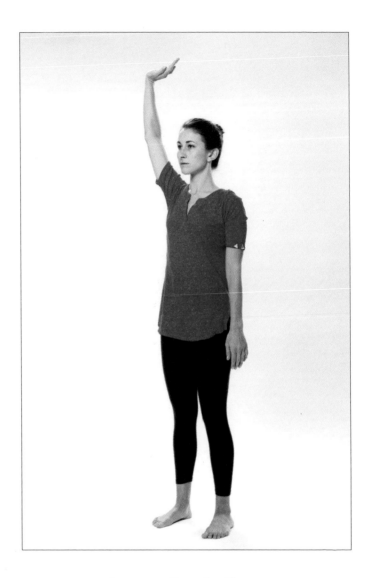

Energy Freely Rising

Stand with one arm hanging relaxed at your side and the other arm raised to one side above the shoulder. Bend your wrist so your palm faces the ceiling and your elbow is straight. Hold and then release. Repeat on both sides. Then relax your arms and stand still.

Group Four

Expanding Wholeness

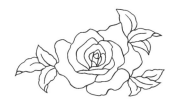

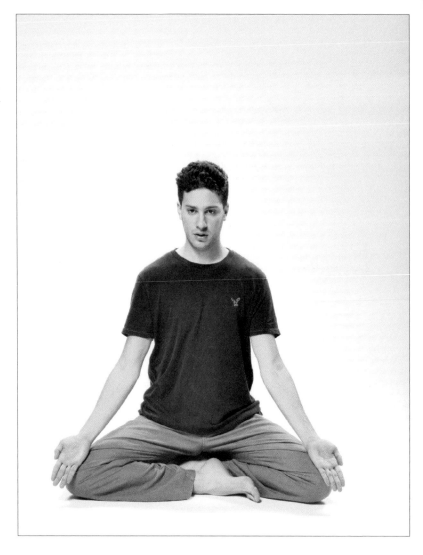

Releasing Positions - *Step One*

Take a comfortable sitting posture with your back straight and your chin tucked in slightly. Place your hands on your knees and open them, palm outward. Relax your arms completely and feel the energy flow from shoulder to hand.

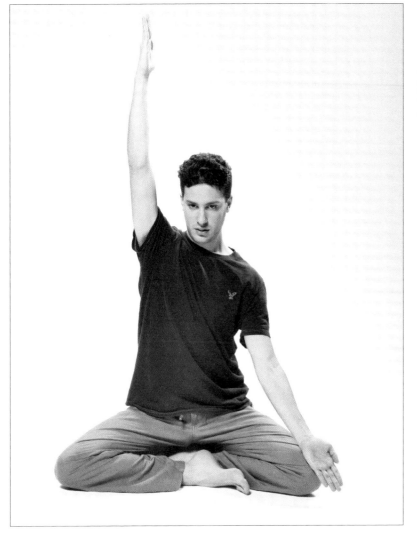

Releasing Positions - *Step Two*

Then raise one arm up straight along the side of your head, leaving the palm extended and facing in toward the body. Leave the other hand extended palm out on your knee. Hold this position a while.

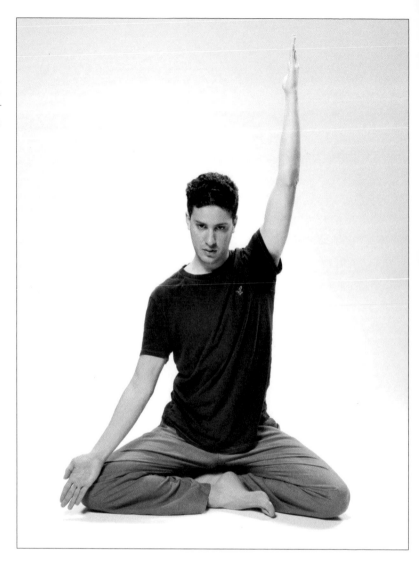

Releasing Positions - Step Three

Then lower the extended arm and return that hand to the knee, leaving it palm up, and bring the other arm up straight along the other side of your head. Hold that position a while.

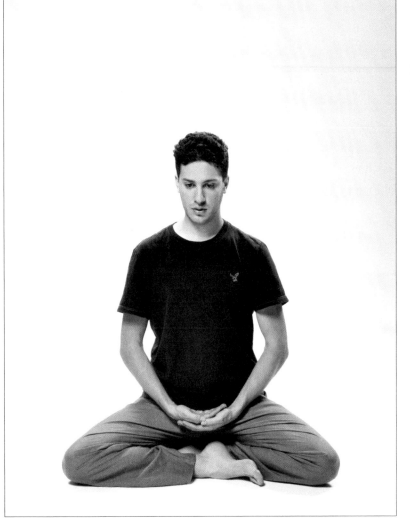

Releasing Positions - Step Four

Lower the extended arm and bring that hand to the knee leaving it palm up. Conclude by cradling the hands together resting on your crossed legs. Let the energy in the upper body completely melt and flow into space.

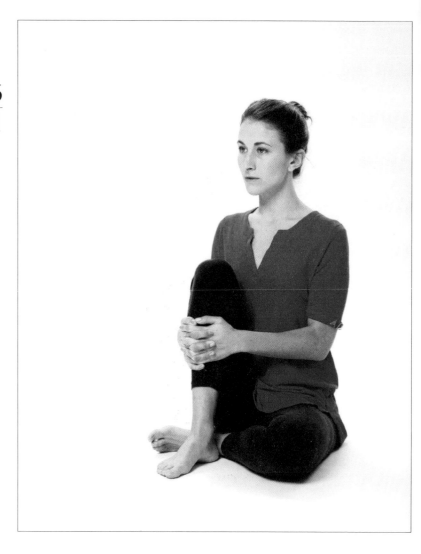

Body of Rhythm - Step One

Take a sitting posture, preferably on a cushion. Pull one knee up to your chest and hold it close to your body. As you hold this posture, contract and condense your energy. Then extend the leg completely, while expanding and lightening your energy.

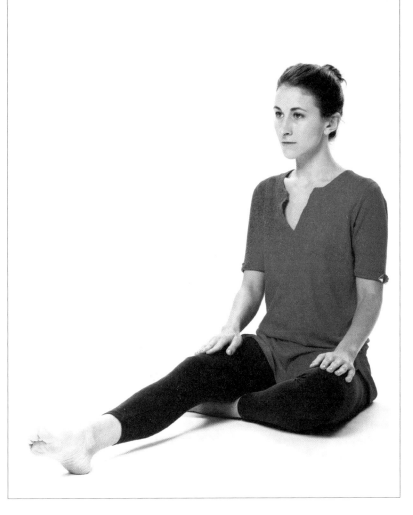

Body of Rhythm - *Step Two*

Do this several times, with each knee separately, paying attention to the beginning, middle, and end of each
movement.

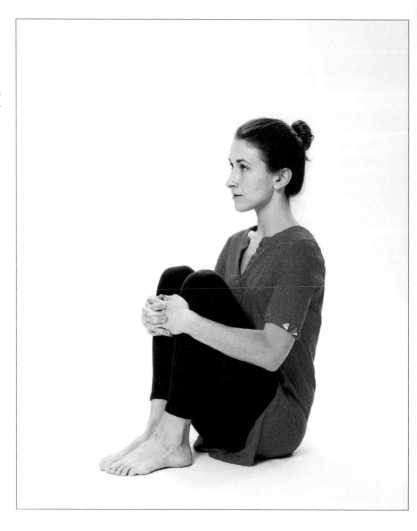

Body of Rhythm - Step Three

Then pull both knees together up close to the body while leaving your feet flat on the floor. Stay in touch with your sense of stability and groundedness.

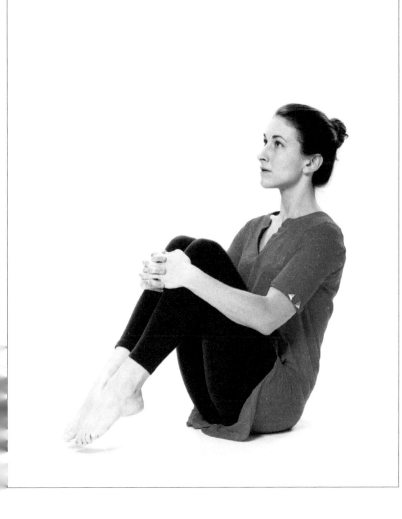

Body of Rhythm - Step Four

Lift your feet off the floor and let your body rock backward. Then bring it forward and backward again. Start with a very small rocking motion. Try keeping your feet off the floor throughout the forward and backward motion. When you come to a stop, put your feet on the floor again, and let everything be completely still.

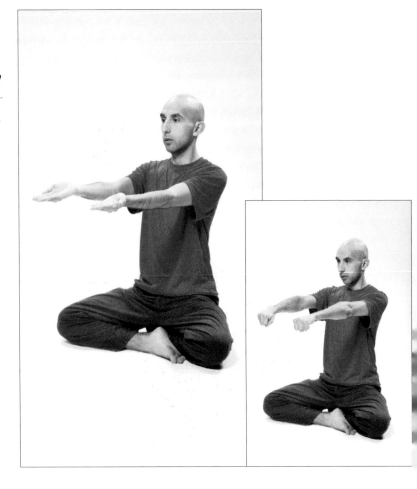

Awakening Heart - Step One

Sit with your arms extended in front of you with the palms facing up. Then make tight fists and rotate the wrists so the fists are facing down. Feel the energy of your hands and the sensations throughout the entire length of your arms. Then bring the fists together in front of your heart, fists still facing down, with the elbows bent.

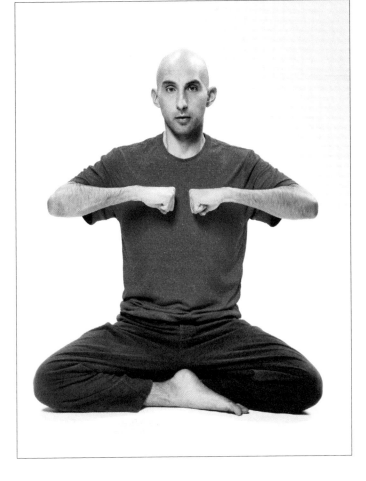

Awakening Heart - Step Two

Without raising your shoulders, and keeping the elbows square to the floor, push the energy of each fist intensely into the other, without letting the fists physically touch. After a little while, place the hands down on the knees and focus into the energy in the chest. Repeat three times.

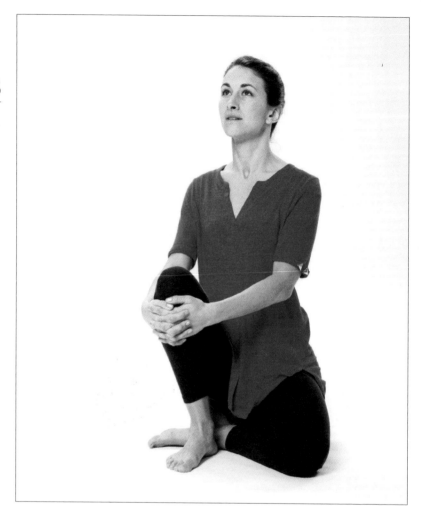

Exercising Flexibility - Step One

Sit with one knee drawn up to the chest and the other in the half-lotus position. Keep the back straight but tilt the head just slightly backward. Grasp the knee with both hands and push the belly out strongly. Hold this posture a while.

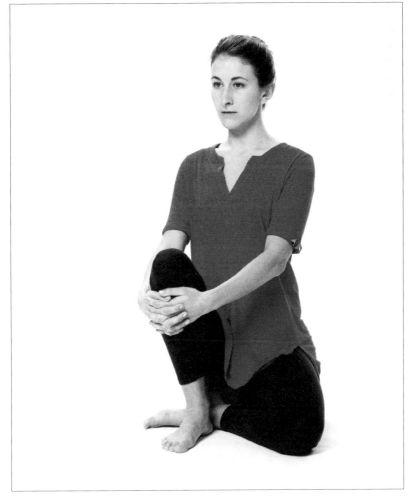

Exercising Flexibility - Step Two

Pull the chest up, straighten the back, pull the chin in slightly, and tighten the belly strongly. Hold this posture. Then shift back to the first posture. Repeat these two postures three times. Then relax and float, as if in water. Switch to the other side and repeat the two postures three times again, ending with floating.

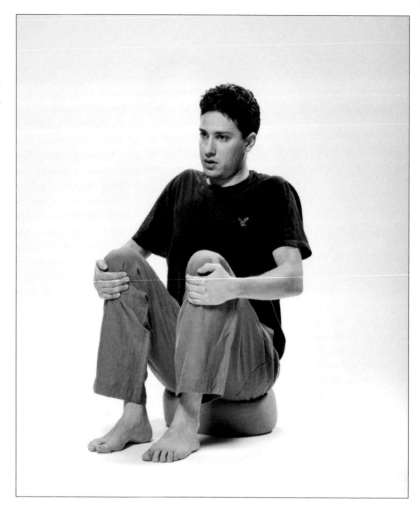

Being in Time - Step One

Sit with both hands around both knees. Push the shoulders up a little higher and pull in the belly. Leave the mouth open and let the breath be. Keep the back straight and push the belly in tight as if it were touching the spine. Loosen the neck and throat, and feel the air in the chest.

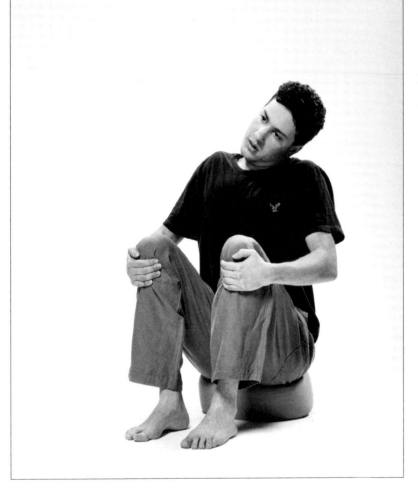

Being in Time - Step Two

Now continue to keep the belly clenched tight and the breath flowing naturally, and tilt the head from side to side, without moving the upper body. Leave the shoulders pulled up and straight as you tilt the head several times to each side. Then bring the head to center and release the belly. Sit completely still and feel the flow of breath in time.

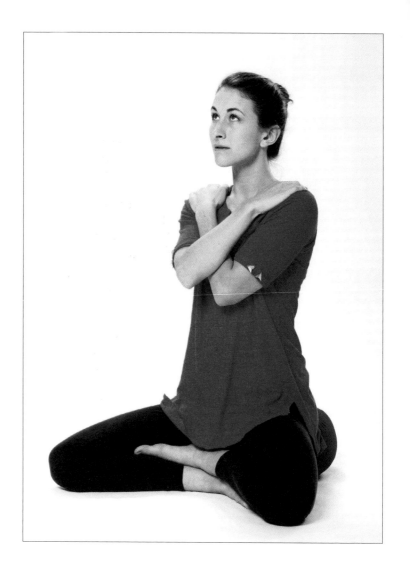

Transparent Wholeness - Step One

Sit with arms folded across chest, hands on your shoulders
so both elbows almost overlap in front of your chest. Look
up but do not tilt the head up. Gently let yourself notice
that everything within the mind and body, sensations, feelings, thoughts, images, is light and empty. Then return to
the seven gestures.

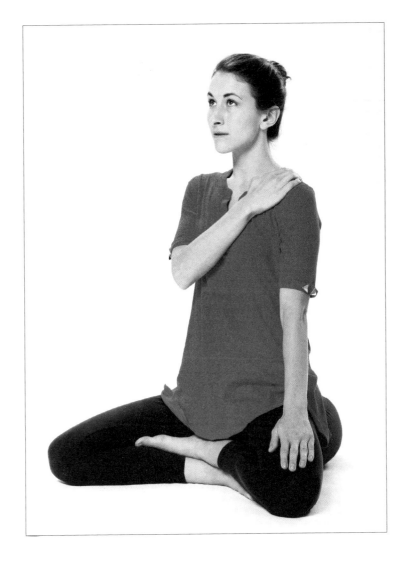

Transparent Wholeness - *Step Two*

Then bring one hand across chest and rest that hand on the opposite shoulder. Leave the other hand resting upon the knee.

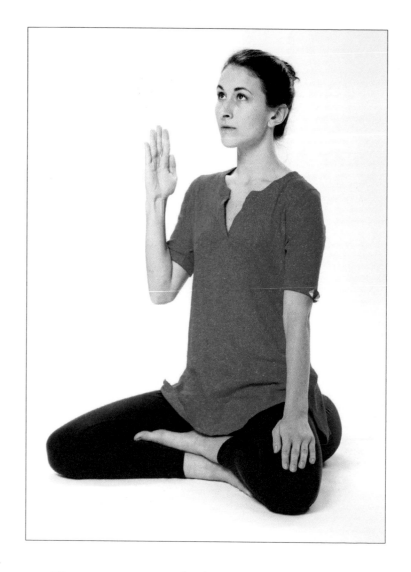

Transparent Wholeness - Step Three

Bring your arm back down to your side with your elbow bent. Pause in this position. Then extend the arm straight up along side of your head until the elbow is straightened out. Let the eyes remain looking up. Hold the position.

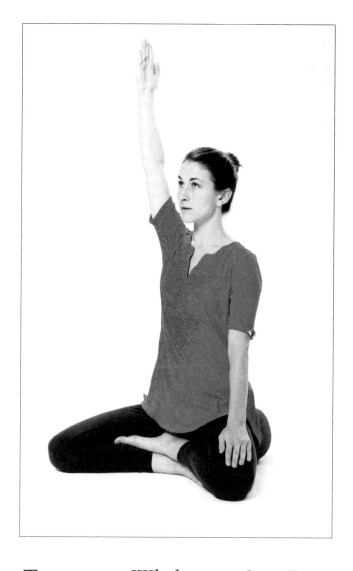

Transparent Wholeness - Step Four
Repeat this extending and bending three times. Then switch to the other side and do three cycles. Finish in the lotus posture with hands on your knees, eyes relaxed, and just gently be.

Group Five

Harmonizing

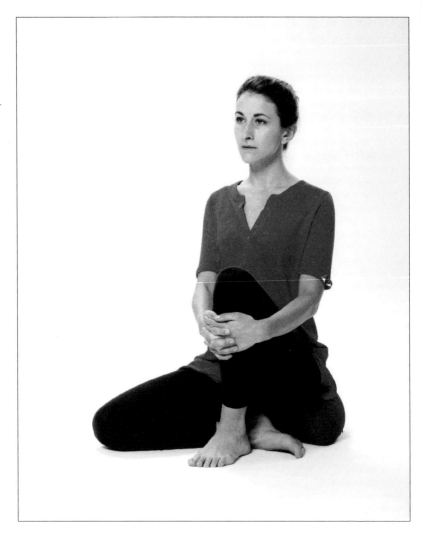

Balancing Inner & Outer - Step One

Sit in the half-lotus posture on a cushion. Then bring one knee up close to your chest and wrap both hands around it. Leave your shoulders relaxed, and keep your neck gently straight. Feel the quality of being completely stable and balanced, focusing especially on your connection with the ground.

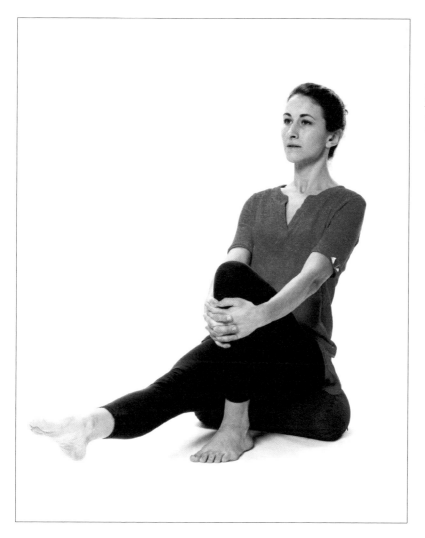

Balancing Inner & Outer - Step Two

Lean back a little and raise the other leg out straight, lifting it up parallel to the floor or as close as you can hold it to parallel. Hold the posture and focus on your inner center of gravity. Repeat three times on each side.

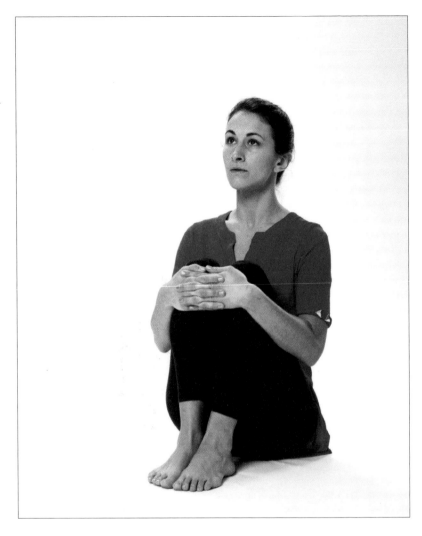

Balancing Inner & Outer - Step Three

Sit directly on the floor or remain on the cushion with your knees drawn up together in front of your chest. Wrap both hands around the knees, interlacing your fingers. Let the clasped hands pull the knees toward the chest without the feet leaving the floor. Gaze gently upward and feel the energy along the spine and your body contacting the ground.

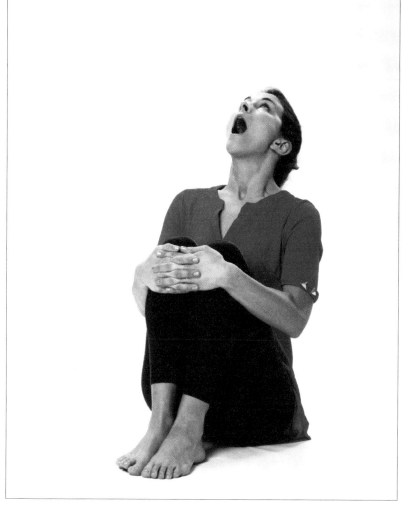

Balancing Inner & Outer - Step Four

Lean back gently, pushing the chest back, and keeping the chin tucked gently in, with your face pointing toward the ceiling. Look up and let the mouth be wide open for a few minutes. Return to the half-lotus posture and sit quietly for a little while.

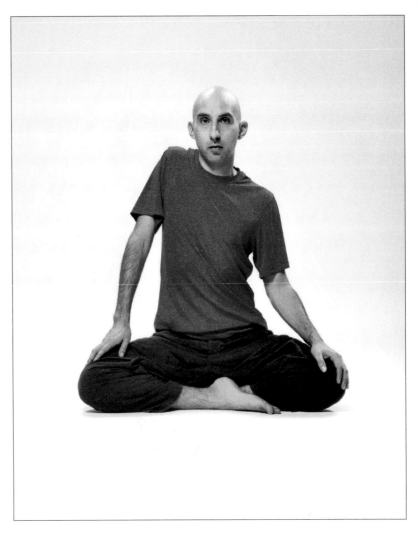

Harmonizing Opposites - Step One

Sit half-lotus style with your hands on your knees. Push one shoulder up and rotate it around from front to back and from back to front. Then do the same with the other shoulder. Leave your neck relaxed and straight. Do this three times on each side.

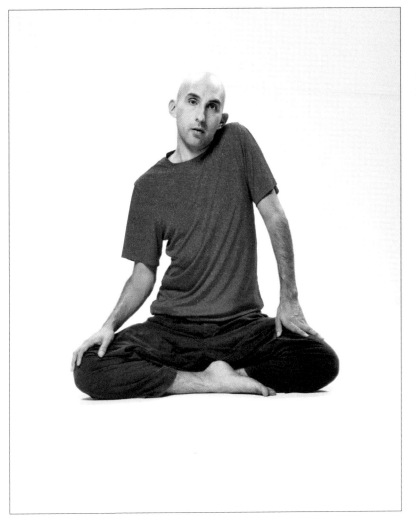

Harmonizing Opposites - Step Two

Now repeat the shoulder raise, and let your head follow as each shoulder goes up. Tilt your head to that side and gently stretch the other side of the neck. Keep your back very straight but let your belly be loose. Repeat several times on each side.

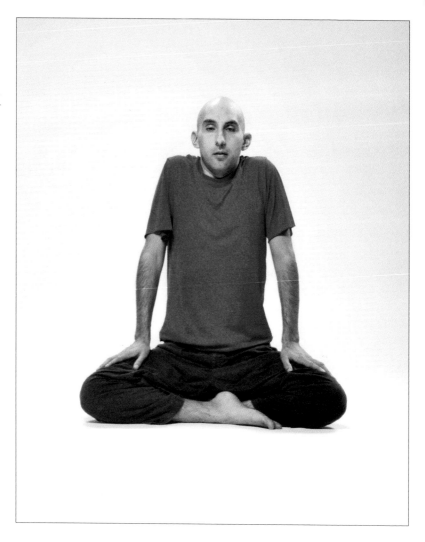

Harmonizing Opposites - Step Three

Now tighten your belly and keep your back straight and strong. Raise both shoulders a little bit and tighten them. Hold this posture a little while. Then exhale slowly and relax.

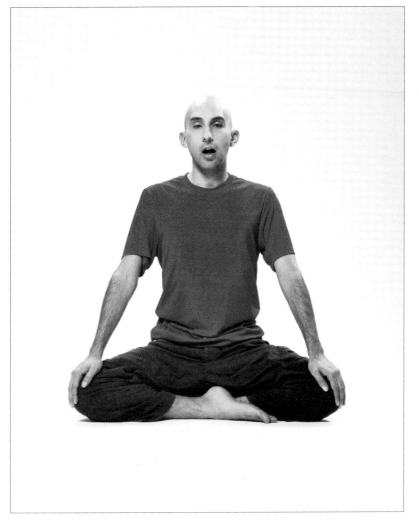

Letting Go Images

Take a sitting posture with your palms on your knees. Let the arms be straight, the hands straight, and the back straight. Feel the strength of the posture. Breathe out slowly, AAH AAH. The fi rst exhale is strong. The second exhale is gentlc. Sit quietly.

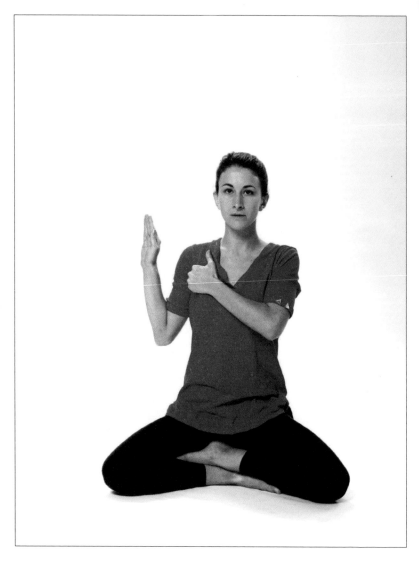

Releasing Resistance - Step One

Take a sitting posture or standing posture. Stretch one arm out to the side, palm facing out, and tuck the other into the armpit. Bend your arm at the elbow, and pull the arm straight back, leaving the hand facing out.

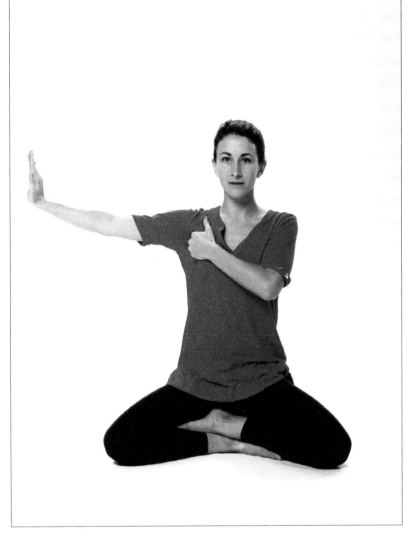

Releasing Resistance - Step Two

Then stretch your arm out again, with the palm outward, pushing space. Repeat three times on each side.

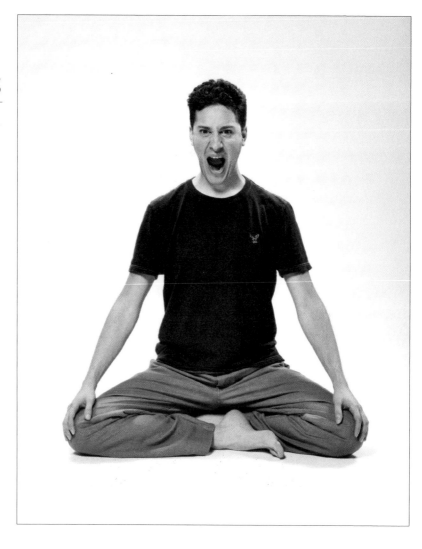

Vibrant Harmony - Step One

Sit in the posture of the Seven Gestures. Make a fierce grin and exaggerate the gesture. Tighten your neck muscles and feel the tension in your face and neck. Hold the expression for a little while.

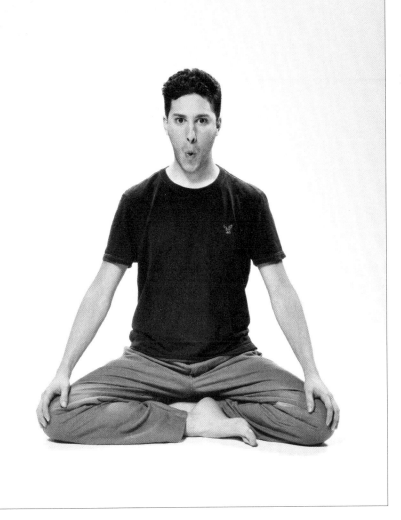

Vibrant Harmony - Step Two

Then make a small circle with your lips brought very strong-ly together and your eyes wide open and round. Feel the tension in your face and neck. Hold the expres-sion. Switch back and forth several times between the two expressions.

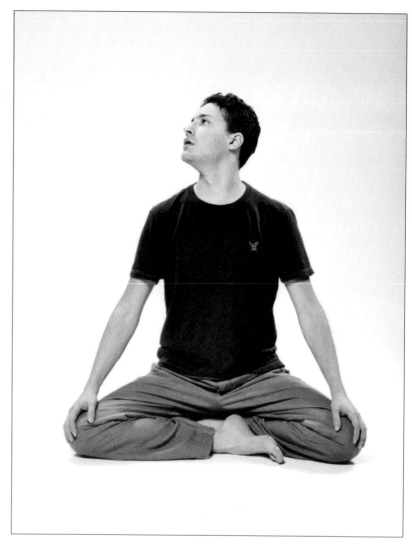

Vibrant Harmony - Step Three

Tilt the chin up to one side and move gently back and forth. Repeat on the other side. Exhale strongly. Sit quietly and feel the energy flow, especially in the throat.

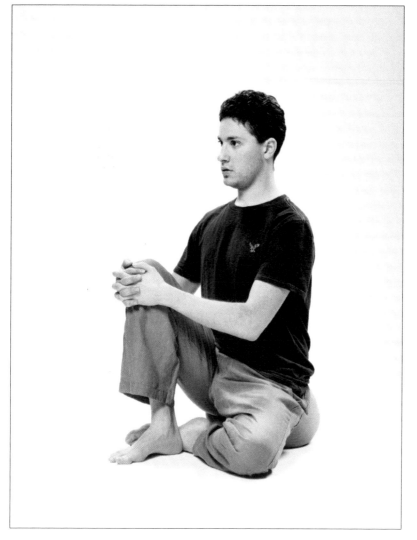

Relinquishing Negativity - Step One

Take a sitting posture with one knee brought up close to chest. Lock your hands around your knee and keep that foot in close to the body.

Relinquishing Negativity - *Step Two*
Straighten your back and then gently lean backward, letting
your head arch backward. Repeat the same gestures with the
other knee.

Group Six

Opening Presence

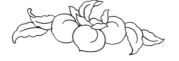

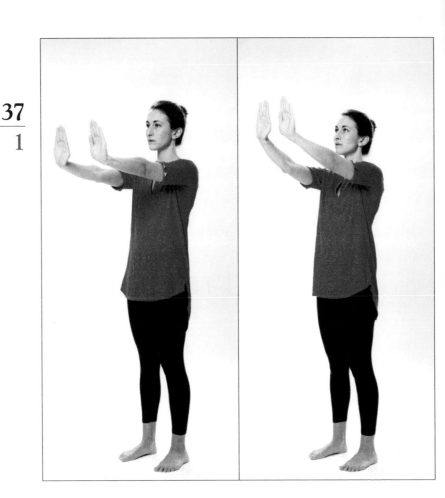

Opening Mind & Body - Step One

Stand with your feet about five inches apart. Stretch your arms out in front of you, with hands at eye level, palms facing out and fingers pointing up. Move your chin a little forward, and raise your shoulders up a bit. Let your eyes gaze toward the top of your fingers. Feel the energy flow in the neck and back, and gently connect those sensations through your shoulders into your arms.

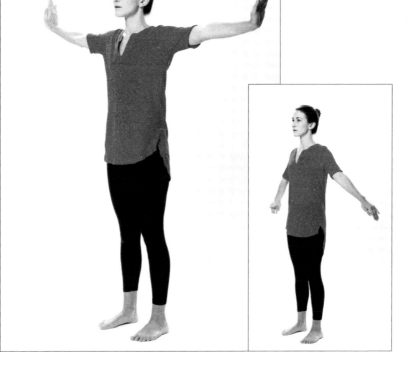

Opening Mind & Body - *Step Two*

Then move your hands apart until your arms are spread
out to the sides at shoulder height. Hold for a while. Then
lower arms with palms in toward the body. Repeat several
times. Pay attention to the sensations in the shoulders, elbows, and wrists and the flow of feeling in the chest. As you
lower your arms, stay closely in touch with the sensations in
the lower body as well.

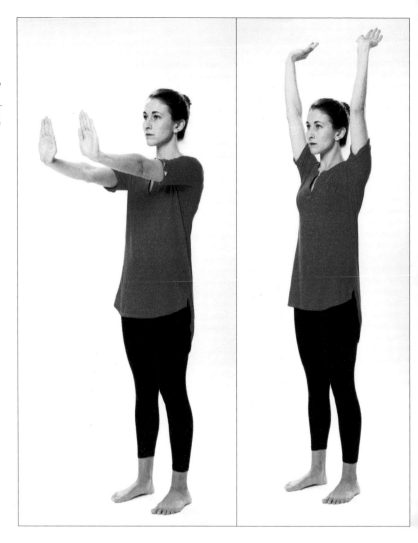

Opening Mind & Body - Step Three

Stand with your arms stretched out in front of you with hands held palms out and fingers pointing up. Then raise your arms until your hands are above your head, with palms still facing out.

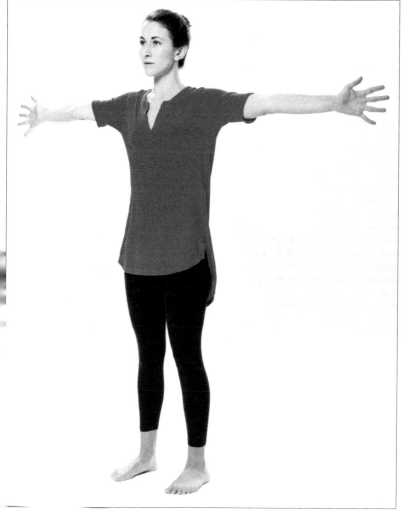

Opening Mind & Body - *Step Four*

Then bring your arms down to shoulder height and stretch your fingers out widely, touching air and space. Gently breathe, mixing sensations into feelings.

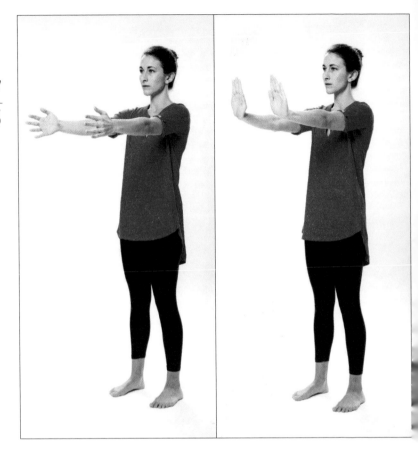

Opening Mind & Body - Step Five

Keep the arms at shoulder height but move them forward until they are extended in fron of you. Bend the wrists, turn the palms outward, and hold the position. Stay in touch with the energy of the shoulders and arms, the back of the neck, and the spine.

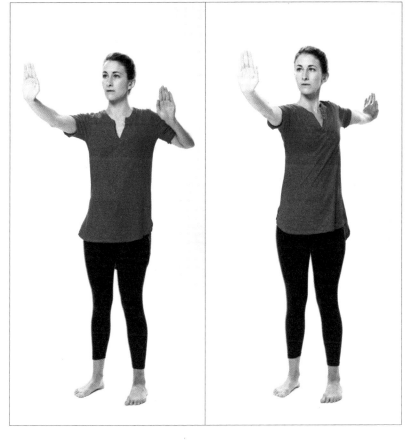

Opening Mind & Body - *Step Six*

Then draw one arm back past your head, leaving the palm turned outward. Feel the tension in the shoulders as you push one arm forward and pull one arm back. Leave the feet in place but let the hips rotate so that you can turn the shoulder, arm, and hand all the way around to let the hand face backward. Then switch sides and repeat.

At first, repeat these six postures in sequence softly and gently. When you become more experienced, you can practice the whole series with more vigor.

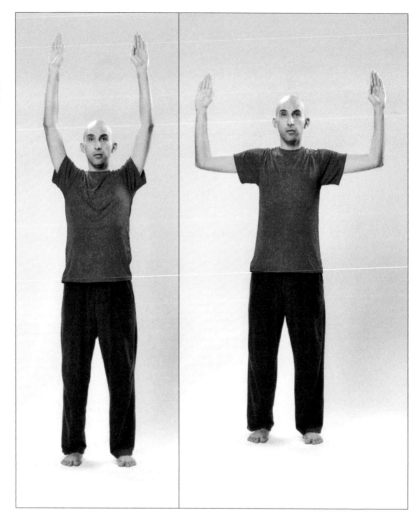

Releasing Beauty - Step One

Stand with your arms raised above your head, with palms facing out. Bend your arms at the elbows and bring your hands down until elbows are square with the floor. Loosen the chest and throat and always breathe gently.

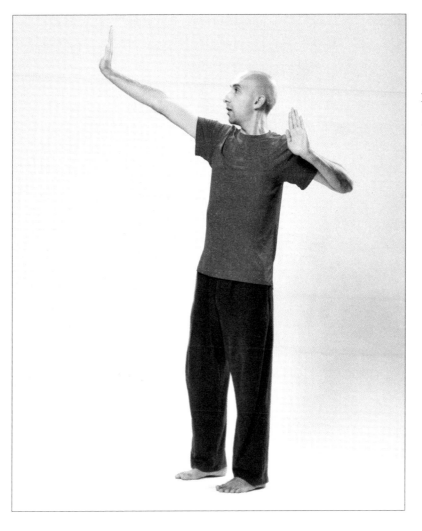

Releasing Beauty - Step Two

Then bring one arm back, keeping the elbow bent and the palm out, and extend one arm forward with the palm out until the elbow is straightened. Keep your face forward. Hold the position a while and then release with arms at your sides. Reverse the position and repeat.

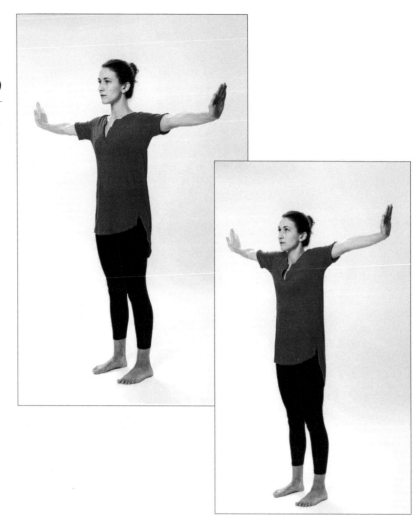

Expanding Joy - Step One

Stand with your arms held out to both sides at shoulder height. Straighten the elbow and flex the wrist so that the palm is perpendicular to floor. Then raise the shoulders and feel the sensations in the chest.

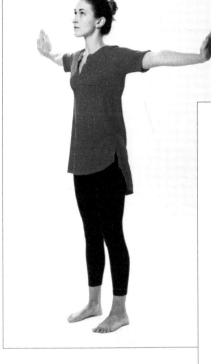

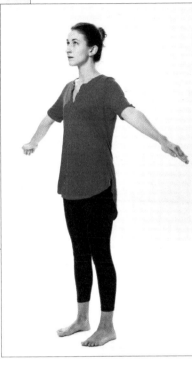

Expanding Joy - *Step Two*

Tighten the back muscles, pulling both sides in toward spine, and let the arms move back. Leave the palms facing out. Tilt the head up slightly and hold the position for a while. Then release the arms slowly and stand still.

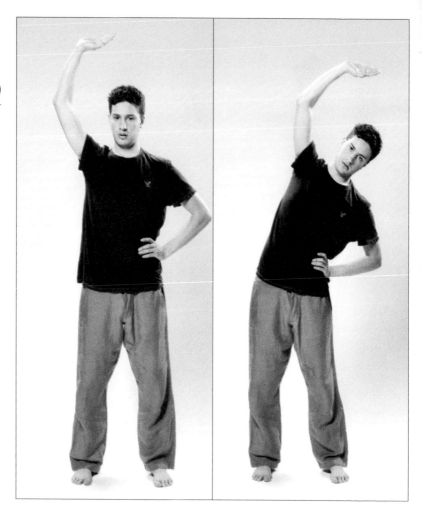

Flowing into Space - Step One

Stand with one hand on the hip and the other raised over the head in a big arc with the palm facing the sky. Keep the face forward and tilt toward the side where hand is on hip. Feel the energy flow through the arched side of body. Then repeat on other side.

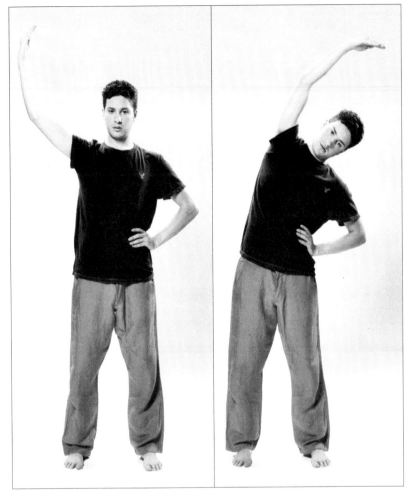

Flowing into Space - Step Two

Leaving one hand on the hip, raise the other arm again, bringing it all the way over the head in a big arc and bending the body to one side slowly. Feel the stretching on the extended side as you slowly bend as far as you can. Keep your face and chest forward. Hold the position for a little while. Then repeat on the other side. Finish by standing still with arms at your sides.

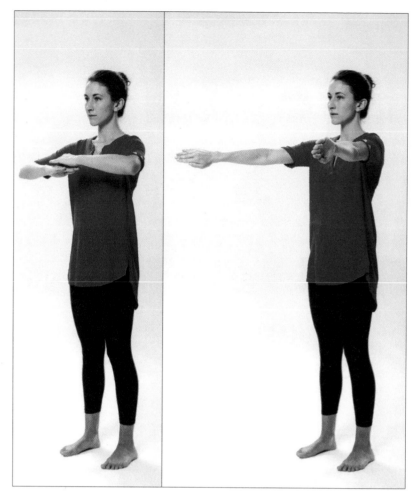

Evoking Presence - Step One

Stand with your arms bent at the elbows and your hands overlapped, but not touching, with both palms down at chest level. Note the energy field between the hands. Then slowly but with strong force, extend the arms out from the elbows and bring them back together. Keep the chest lifted up and the stomach tucked in.

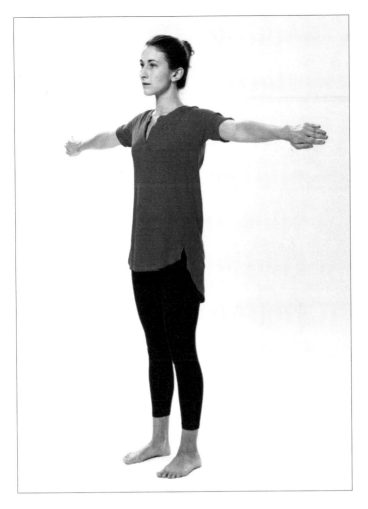

Evoking Presence - Step Two

As you engage Step One and Two, note the wholeness of the body: the parts that are not moving are fully participating in the movement. Note the merging of mind and body as awareness permeates the movements. And note the intimacy of inner and outer as arms open an invisible curtain into the heart of space.

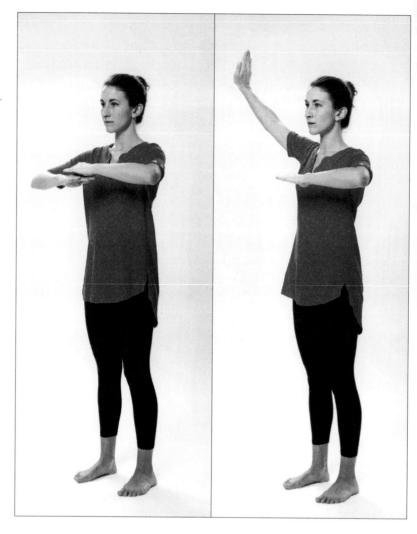

Evoking Presence - Step Three

Return to the position of Step One and then move one arm up over the head, keeping your elbow straight and your palm out. Leave the other arm bent at the elbow, palm down in front of the chest at heart level.

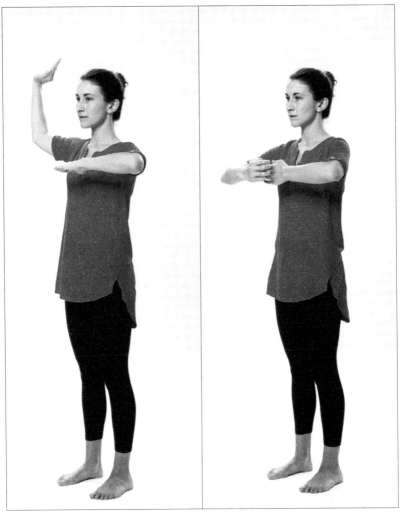

Evoking Presence - Step Four

Bring the raised arm down, bending it at the elbow, and leaving the palm turned up. Hold this posture a while.Note the sensations in the upper chest. Then bring both arms down together facing the chest at heart level, palms in and overlapping. Repeat on the other side.

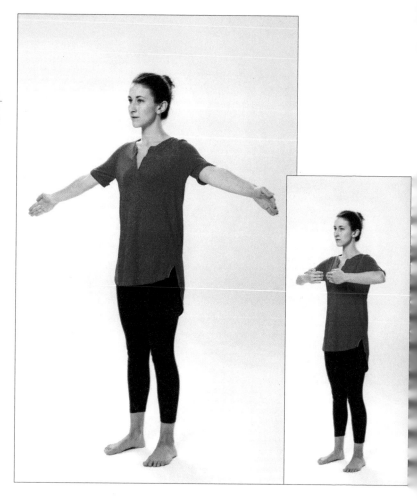

Evoking Presence - Step Five

Move both arms out to the sides of the body, palms facing forward. Then bring both arms back facing the chest at heart level, palms in and fingers nearly touching.

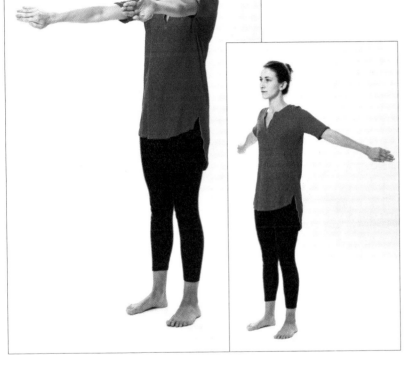

Evoking Presence - Step Six

Rotate both hands at the wrists until the palms are facing outward. Very slowly move the arms out to the sides, as if you were pushing against a powerful force until both arms are extended back with elbows straight. Keep the wrists flexed and the palms facing out throughout the entire movement. Hold this posture a little while.

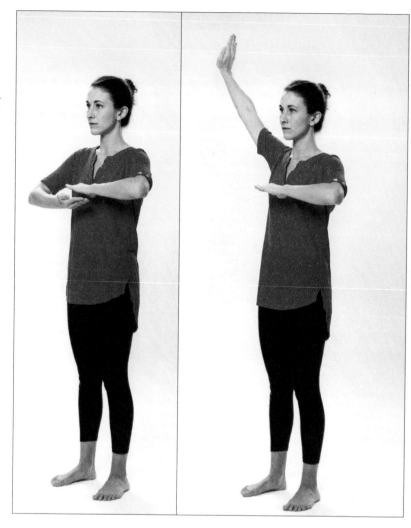

Evoking Presence - Step Seven

Bring your arms together again at heart level, overlapping with lower palm facing up and upper palm facing down. Raise one arm up with the palm out and wrist flexed, and the elbow straight. Then bring the arm back down to the heart level. Repeat on the other side.

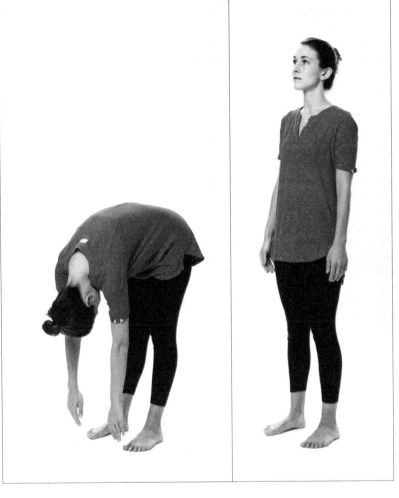

Evoking Presence - *Step Eight*

Bend over at the waist, and let the neck relax and the head hang down loosely. Move the chin forward and release air. Hold this position for a moment. Then gently return to a standing position and deeply relax into vividly present energy.

Index

294

Flowing into Space (#40),
284-285
focus, 3, 23, 30
  sustain, 42
forbearance, 63
form/s,
  How our bodies took, 7
  of existence, 7
fortunate
  aeon, 151
  realms, 66
foundation/s, xiv, 3, 18, 31, 40,
47, 54, 58, 61-63, 85, 94, 111,
131, 150, 154, 164-166, 168, 179
  essential 21
  for enlightenment, 54
  for satisfaction & joy, 61
  of knowledge, 111
  of mindfulness, 150
  a sound/balanced, 7, 154
four,
  Bases of spiritual powers,
  150
  Foundations of
  mindfulness, 150
fragrance, xvii, 2, 57, 102-103
  and Feeling, 103
  exquisite, 2
  subtleties of, xvii
free, 5, 29, 34, 138, 149
  of doubts, 34
  of fixations, 29
  flow of feeling, 138
  of neediness, 5
Freeing Energy (#3), 196-197

friend,
  Making Mind our, 152-159
  to self and others, 6
frustration/s, xviii, 6, 38, 153
fulfilling, 5, 17
fully, 5-6, 53, 57, 151
fundamental,
  human expressions, 90
  minds, 7
  of pressures, the most 153
  structures, 7
Gampopa, 163
gates to meaning, 72
gateway, 62
  opening, 3
  to Meditation, 184
General Guidelines for
  Exercises, 193
Generating Happiness from
  Within, 61
generosity,
  joy inspires, xvi
  of heart, xvi
  Confidence that is, xiv
gesture, 22-24, 33
  of gratitude, xviii
Gestures, Seven, 21-26, 36-37,
48, 156, 176, 192, 194, 268
Getting the Juice of
  Experience, 117-134
glowing, 53
good friend, 6, 71, 148
  To yourself, 148
grasping, 19, 36, 104-106, 114,
118, 143, 152

Suggested Readings
on Mind and Mental Events

Mind in Buddhist Psychology
"Necklace of Clear Understanding"
by Yeshe Gyaltsen
Translated by H. V. Guenther and L. S. Kawamura
Dharma Publishing, 1975

Ways of Enlightenment
Buddhist Studies at Nyingma Institute
Based on Lama Mipham's mKhas-'jug
Dharma Publishing, 1993

Gathering the Meanings: Essential Teachings of the Buddha
The Arthaviniscaya Sutra and its Commentary, Nibandhana
Translated by N. H. Samtani

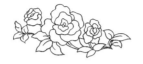

Kum Nye Tibetan Yoga

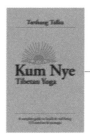

A complete guide to health & wellbeing; 115 exercises & massages

Based on a traditional healing system, Kum Nye Yoga helps to relieve stress, transform negative patterns and promote balance and health. The practice of Kum Nye increases our enjoyment and appreciation of life.

The unique value of this Tibetan healing system is that it integrates the physical and psychological approaches to wellbeing, teaching us to integrate body and mind in all our activities. Kum Nye leads to a sense of vitality and wellness beyond what can be experienced in other physical systems of exercise. Its postures and movements as well as its self-massage and breathing practices relax the body, calm the breath and still the mind, making this type of yoga an effective practice for deepening meditation.

Kum Nye Yoga introduces us to the power and beauty of the spiritual path. Based on Tibetan teachings for living in harmony with physical and universal laws, this practice develops our ability to heal and energize our entire being. Kum Nye Yoga teaches us what it means to just be.

"The key to both internal integration and a balanced relationship with the world lies within our feelings and sensations. We can nurture and heal both our body and mind by touching our feelings deeply and expand the flowing rhythms they bring to us, for they are linked to the vitality of the universe itself."

ISBN 978-0-89800-421-2 / 425 pp. / $26.00

Kum Nye Dancing

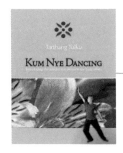

Introducing Mind to the Treasures the Body Offers

"The exercises in this book are new. These are not traditional Kum Nye postures, but instead are based on temple practices I had learned as a young man in Tibet. I drew upon my recollections of exercises that prepare lamas for the sacred ritual movement colloquially known as lama dancing. Traditional lama dancing uses physical choreography to open up the self and liberate energy for Dharma activity; these exercises, intensifying feeling in similar ways, can tame resistance, resentment, and lack of cooperation. The practices in this book are invigorating rather than soothing, designed to energize the body and to wake up consciousness."

Tarthang Tulku, *Kum Nye Dancing* – Introduction

Kum Nye is the art of making friends with all experience. When we practice the gestures, we become familiar with the body's subtle flows of energy. Through movement, energy expresses meaning and liberates the mind. Dynamic and expressive, the Kum Nye Dancing postures manifest the understanding that only in the present moment can we find real nourishment and knowledge. These postures ignite the power to engage us now.

ISBN 978-0-89800-006-1 / 220 pp. / $25.00

Kum Nye Programs

Wellness and Wholeness

Kum Nye yoga is a gentle healing system that relieves stress, transforms negative patterns, and helps us to be balanced and healthy. Kum Nye yoga relaxes the senses and heals the constricting patterns of behavior and attitude, balancing, integrating and energizing the whole of our being; a foundation of inner wellness that improves the quality of all interactions with the world around us.

The Art of Balance

The key to balance lies within our feelings and sensations. We can nurture and heal our bodies and minds by touching our feelings deeply and expanding their flowing rhythms that are linked to the energy of the universe itself. This energy can stimulate itself internally, recycling residues of emotional patterns and making us alive and well.

Kum Nye Yoga

Kum (Tibetan: sKu) refers to the body. It refers not so much to the physical body, rather to our human embodiment, our embodied, authentic existence. Kum encompasses all aspects of our being.

Nye (Tibetan: mNye) means internal massage of life's energies or the feelings in the body. It refines, recreates, and regenerates all the patterns of living. With Nye, our energy constantly refreshes itself.

Yoga refers to integration; with Kum Nye yoga life's energies become integrated and we experience internal wellness and external wholeness. Practicing the nine levels of Kum Nye yoga refines the inner architecture of our subtle body energy system.

Kum Nye - Gateway to Enlightened Vision: Kum Nye exercises generate a relaxing process of body and mind that opens a path of spiritual development in the midst of daily life, laying a foundation for meditative practices. In calm and relaxed states of well-being, there naturally arises the knowledge and strength we need.

Kum Nye Lineage: Introduced by Tarthang Tulku in the early 1970's, Kum Nye is a living tradition that Dharma Publishing offers in four books: Kum Nye: A Tibetan Yoga (formerly Kum Nye Relaxation Vol. I and II); Tibetan Relaxation; The Joy of Being; and Kum Nye Dancing. Kum Nye is available on Audio CDs, DVDs and by eKum Nye.

"Kum Nye practices are symbols, pointing to the nature of all existence."

Tarthang Tulku

eKum Nye is a program by email, directly from Dharma Publishing Programs. Offered in English, Dutch, German, Spanish and Portuguese, this e-program is a step-by-step guide to deepen your practice of Kum Nye Yoga and your understanding of how to live in accord with its basic principles.

eKum Nye Yoga consists of the basic Five Levels, each level structured in ten weekly segments. After finishing Level I, one proceeds to Level II, and so on. All together, the Five Levels of Kum Nye Yoga by email provide a year-long intensive Kum Nye training. Additional levels are available, such as The Top Ten; Kum Nye in a Nutshell (five segments: Opening, Healing, Stimulating, Manifesting and Protecting); and Speech and Mind Kum Nye.

The Five Levels of eKum Nye Yoga:
1. Outer Kum Nye Relaxation: Opening to feeling and to the energy of the breath.
2. Transformations: Wholeness through stimulating and transforming energies.
3. Inner Balance: Integrating body and mind to engender wellness.
4. Cream of Kum Nye: Advanced Kum Nye to liberate the senses and mind.
5. Extracting the Juice of Experience: the Joy of Being.
Each class contains: Kum Nye theory, two short videos, five-minute meditations, a practice session of 60 - 90 minutes, and reading assignments.

Additional eKum Nye topics:
6. Top Ten Kum Nye Exercises: ten lessons with theory, recommendations, questions and answers.
7. Power of Breath: eleven lessons on the healing and stimulating power of the breath.
8. Kum Nye in a Nutshell: five segments, Opening, Healing, Stimulating, Manifesting, Protecting.
9. Speech and Mind Kum Nye: ten lessons to begin undoing the labeling of past experiences and learning to relax the one who is doing the exercises.
10. Kum Nye in Daily Life: Twelve lessons to sustain the Kum Nye experience in daily life.
11. Generating Happiness

For more information please visit us at www.dharmapublishing.com or email us at programs@dharmapublishing.com

Kum Nye Products
Kum Nye Dancing Series DVDs

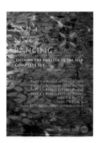

**Opening the
Nucleus of Self**

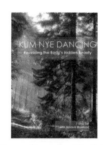

**Revealing the Body's
Hidden Beauty +
Commentary Set**

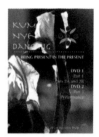

**Being Present
in the Present**

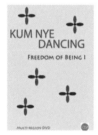

**Freedom of
Being "I"**

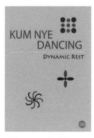

Dynamic Rest

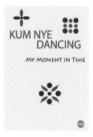

**My Moment
in Time**

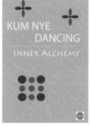

Inner Alchemy

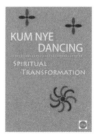

**Spiritual
Transformation**

Kum Nye Products
Kum Nye CDs and Audiobooks

Audiobooks: Audio/MP3 CDs

Kum Nye - Tibetan Yoga
By Tarthang Tulku.
The Audiobook does not contain the exercises.

The Joy of Being:
Advanced Kum Nye Practices
By Tarthang Tulku.
The Audiobook does not contain the exercises.

Kum Nye Relaxation Audio CDs

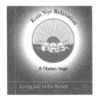

01 Introduction
02 The Art of Developing Balance
03 Integrating Body & Mind
04 Living Life in the Breath
05 Developing Wholeness of Energy
06 Tools for Transformation
07 Healing the Four Energy Centers
08 Stimulating & Transforming Energies
09 Morning and Evening Practices
10 Transmuting Negative Energies

Kum Nye Products

Kum Nye Talks Audio CDs

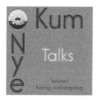

This series features talks with Arnaud Maitland and residential Kum Nye
students at the Ratna Ling Retreat Center.

Volume 1: Feeling & Integrating
Volume 2: Guiding Practice
Volume 3: The Energy of Breath in Kum Nye
Volume 4: Stimulating and Transforming Energies
Volume 5: Kum Nye in Three Books
Volume 6: Introduction to Power Kum Nye
Volume 7: "Kum" & "Nye" in Kum Nye Dancing

Audios are available for download at www.dharmapublishing.com

Kum Nye: Healthy Body and Mind Series

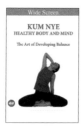 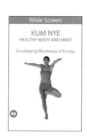 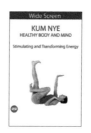 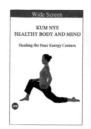

The Art of
Developing
Balance

Developing
Wholeness
of Energy

Stimulating and
Transforming
Energy

Healing the
Four Energy
Centers

Authorized Kum Nye Centers

**Dharma Publishing
Academy**
35788 Hauser Bridge Road
Cazadero, California 95421
(707) 847-3717
www.dharmapublishing.com

Nyingma Centrum Holland
Reguliersgracht 25
1017 LJ Amsterdam
Netherlands
(0031-20) 620-5207
www.nyingma.nl

Instituto Nyingma do Brasil
Rua Cayowáa, 2.085
Sumaré–CEP 01258-011
São Paulo, Brazil
(011) 3864-4785
www.nyingma.com.br

Kum Nye Argentina
www.kumnyeyoga.com.ar

Nyingma Institute
1815 Highland Place
Berkeley, California 94709
(510) 843-6812
www.nyingmainstitute.com

**Nyingma Zentrum
Deutschland**
Siebachstr. 66
50733 Köln
Germany
(0049-221) 589-0474
www.nyingmazentrum.de

Instituto Nyingma Rio
R. Casuarina, 297 - Casa 2 -
Humaitá CEP 22261-160
Rio de Janeiro, Brazil
(021) 2527-9388 or 2286-8426
www.nyingmario.org.br

Kum Nye United Kingdom
www.kumnyeuk.org

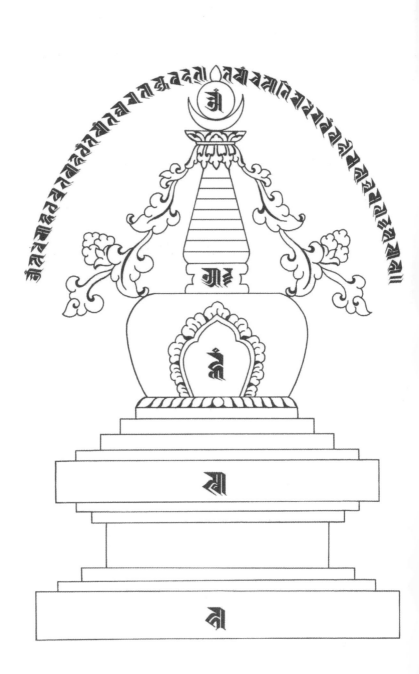